Integrated Primary Care

About the Authors

Barbara Cubic, PhD, has been recognized as a trailblazer for integrated primary care. She has spent her career advocating for psychologists to work in primary care settings and has trained and mentored hundreds of other professionals to do so. In 2010, she was awarded the PSYCHE prize by the American Psychological Foundation for her work in integrated primary care. She has also been awarded the Outstanding Contributions to Clinical Health Psychology award from the Society of Health Psychology of the American Psychological Association in 2014 and the Ivan Mensch Award for Distinguished Achievement in Teaching by the Association of Psychologist in Academic Health Centers in 2017.

Ruben Tinajero, PhD, is a clinical health psychologist in the Department of Family Medicine at West Virginia University. He completed his doctoral training at the University of Utah and internship training at the University of Kansas Medical Center. Dr. Tinajero contributes to the training of WVU family medicine residents and medical school students and supervises doctoral practicum students and psychology interns. His primary research interests are in stress science and sleep research.

Advances in Psychotherapy – Evidence-Based Practice

The basic objective of this series is to provide therapists with practical, evidence-based treatment guidance for the most common disorders seen in clinical practice – and to do so in a reader-friendly manner. Each book in the series is both a compact "how-to" reference on a particular disorder for use by professional clinicians in their daily work and an ideal educational resource for students as well as for practice-oriented continuing education.

The most important feature of the books is that they are practical and easy to use: All are structured similarly and all provide a compact and easy-to-follow guide to all aspects that are relevant in real-life practice. Tables, boxed clinical "pearls," marginal notes, and summary boxes assist orientation, while checklists provide tools for use in daily practice.

Continuing Education Credits

Psychologists and other healthcare providers may earn five continuing education credits for reading the books in the *Advances in Psychotherapy* series and taking a multiple-choice exam. This continuing education program is a partnership of Hogrefe Publishing and the National Register of Health Service Psychologists. Details are available at https://www.hogrefe.com/us/cenatreg

The National Register of Health Service Psychologists is approved by the American Psychological Association to sponsor continuing education for psychologists. The National Register maintains responsibility for this program and its content.

Advances in Psychotherapy – Evidence-Based Practice, Volume 57

Integrated Primary Care

Barbara Cubic
Department of Family Medicine, West Virginia University School of Medicine, Morgantown, WV

Ruben Tinajero
Department of Family Medicine, West Virginia University School of Medicine, Morgantown, WV

hogrefe

Library of Congress Cataloging in Publication information for the print version of this book is available via the Library of Congress Marc Database under the Library of Congress Control Number 2026931560

Library and Archives Canada Cataloguing in Publication
Title: Integrated primary care / Barbara Cubic, Ruben Tinajero, Department of Family Medicine, West Virginia University School of Medicine, Morgantown, WV.
Names: Cubic, Barbara, author. | Tinajero, Ruben author.
Series: Advances in psychotherapy--evidence-based practice ; v. 57.
Description: Series statement: Advances in psychotherapy---evidence-based practice ; volume 57 | Includes bibliographical references.
Identifiers: Canadiana (print) 20250311941 | Canadiana (ebook) 20250315890 | ISBN 9780889376106 (softcover) | ISBN 9781616766108 (PDF) | ISBN 9781613346105 (EPUB)
Subjects: LCSH: Clinical health psychology. | LCSH: Mental health services. | LCSH: Integrated delivery of health care. | LCSH: Primary care (Medicine)
Classification: LCC R726.7 .C83 2026 | DDC 616.001/9—dc23

www.hogrefe.com

Publishing Offices
USA: Hogrefe Publishing Corporation, 44 Merrimac St., Newburyport, MA 01950
Phone 978 255 3700; E-mail customersupport@hogrefe.com
EUROPE: Hogrefe Publishing GmbH, Merkelstr. 3, 37085 Göttingen, Germany
Phone +49 551 99950 0, Fax +49 551 99950 111; E-mail publishing@hogrefe.com

Sales & Distribution
USA: Hogrefe Publishing, Customer Services Department, 30 Amberwood Parkway, Ashland, OH 44805
Phone 800 228 3749, Fax 419 281 6883; E-mail customersupport@hogrefe.com
UK: Hogrefe Ltd, Hogrefe House, Albion Place, Oxford, OX1 1QZ
Phone +44 186 579 7920; E-mail customersupport@hogrefe.co.uk
EUROPE: Hogrefe Publishing, Merkelstr. 3, 37085 Göttingen, Germany
Phone +49 551 99950 0, Fax +49 551 99950 111; E-mail publishing@hogrefe.com

Other Offices
CANADA: Hogrefe Publishing Corporation, 82 Laird Drive, East York, Ontario, M4G 3V1
SWITZERLAND: Hogrefe Publishing, Länggass-Strasse 76, 3012 Bern

Printed and bound in the USA

ISBN 978-0-88937-610-6 (print) • ISBN 978-1-61676-610-8 (PDF) • ISBN 978-1-61334-610-5 (EPUB)
https://doi.org/10.1027/00610-000

Acknowledgments

Our experiences in primary care have strengthened us both personally and professionally. We would like to thank our patients, their families, and the many providers we have had the pleasure of working with in primary care. We would also like to thank our many psychology mentors and the psychology trainees who have trusted us to teach them to operate effectively as psychologists in primary care settings.

Barbara would also like to thank her husband, Bill Adams, and her two beautiful daughters, Sarah and Emily, who inspire her daily to be a better person and psychologist. She would like to thank her sister, Susan Supinger, for always being her biggest cheerleader. And, most of all, she would like to thank her father, Ray May, and paternal grandmother, Hancie May, for teaching her the value of education and the importance of being a caring and compassionate person. She also wants to acknowledge the impact her mentors had on her personal and professional life – most notably, Danny Wedding, Don Williamson, and Judy Beck.

Ruben would like to thank his parents, Ruben C. Tinajero and Hilda A. Tinajero, for a lifetime of love and support. He would also like to thank his wonderful wife, Amber, and beautiful daughter, Lila, who have served as sources of motivation for him each day. He wants, as well, to extend his gratitude to his mentors Paula G. Williams, Katherine T. Fortenberry, Timothy W. Smith, and Annette L. Stanton. Lastly, he would like to thank his late aunt, Alma Rosa Arroyo Navarro, who inspired him to achieve his academic dreams.

Contents

1

Description

1.1 Terminology and Definitions

Primary care (PC) is defined as "the provision of *integrated, accessible* health care services by clinicians who are *accountable* for addressing a large majority of personal health care needs, developing a *sustained* partnership with patients, and practicing in the context of *family and community*" (Institute of Medicine, Committee on the Future of Primary Care, 1994). Typically, PC providers are from the disciplines of family medicine, internal medicine, pediatrics, and sometimes obstetrics and gynecology, as these specialties provide care that is preventative, for acute or chronic conditions, across the spectrum of clinical presentations. These specialties also assist patients in the coordination of referrals as needed, often utilize team-based care models, and have continuous relationships with their patients, at times from birth through end of life. PC practices are embedded in communities and integrally connected with community resources. *Primary care providers* (PCPs) provide services in a variety of health care settings including hospitals, outpatient clinics, critical care settings, long-term facilities, and within patients' homes. In addition to the provision of medical services, PC settings are the most common locations for the provision of behavioral health care. However, PCPs often report being ill-prepared to deal with the behavioral health needs of their patients, and describe this as a point of stress for their practices. In fact, PCPs write prescriptions for psychotropic medications more frequently than any other medical discipline, including psychiatry (Hughes et al., 2024). Because PC is the setting where most patients receive their behavioral health services, it has often been called the de facto mental health system in the United States (Cummings et al., 2001). Patients seen in PC settings for behavioral health needs rarely follow up with specialty mental health providers, despite frequent referrals to do so, which many speculate is due to the stigma associated with obtaining care for mental health needs (Ahad et al., 2023). When surveyed, most patients have reported that they would prefer to receive their behavioral health services in a PC setting because of convenience, lack of stigma, and coordination of care between their PCP and their *behavioral health provider* (BHP; Lang, 2005). The importance of this issue is underscored by the fact that data clearly show that behavioral health issues exacerbate physical health problems and vice versa.

Primary care is generally the first point of care for most individuals utilizing health care

Primary care providers come from a variety of medical specialties

Numerous medical professions are employed within PC settings. In this book, the term "PCP" refers to PC attending physicians, residents, and other *advanced practice providers* (APPs), such as nurse practitioners and physician assistants. Other medical PC team members include medical assistants, nurses, pharmacists, dietitians, and lab technicians, among others. Various BHPs may also be a part of the team if the practice is integrated (*integrated primary care* [IPC]), and these include, but are not limited to, psychologists, psychiatrists, social workers, professional counselors, and mental health technicians. The term "BHP" as used in this book may refer to practitioners from all of these disciplines or only some of them – as indicated. At times, the term BHP and mental health clinician or specialist may be used interchangeably. Also, please note that at times a clinician from a mental health discipline could be in PC but not necessarily be involved in IPC. For example, a social worker could be placed in PC to assist with a discharge clinic but not be available for warm handoffs and other IPC clinical activities.

PC settings utilize a population-based model of care

Providers in PC settings have to take care of the needs of a population of patients, without exceeding allocated resources (e.g., staff, providers, space, equipment, technology). To accomplish this, PC clinics will place a large emphasis on wellness and prevention. Keeping a large majority of individuals physically and mentally healthy within the population allows more time and resources to be allocated toward those who ultimately develop acute or chronic health care concerns. PCPs are also tasked with creating strong patient–provider relationships and maintaining them longitudinally, which enhances their ability to identify health risks and interrupt their impact early. To do so, clinics often screen their patient population for common conditions (e.g., cardiac disease, diabetes, asthma, depression, and anxiety) to support better health care outcomes. For example, screening for depression annually (or more frequently) facilitates mental health interventions that can be offered at the onset of a depressive episode as opposed to once the depression has become entrenched. While PCPs are often adept at offering pharmacological interventions for milder forms of depression or providing brief psychoeducation and counseling, having access to BHPs allows them to offer a patient with depression more comprehensive care. Access to BHPs becomes increasingly important as the severity of a behavioral concern increases. Thus, IPC is needed.

IPC encapsulates care models that utilize medical providers and behavioral health care clinicians working together

Integrated primary and specialty care developed out of the recognition that the fragmentation of the health care system was not accomplishing the goal of creating a healthier population. The volume of patients seen in PC and the variegated needs of these patients could not be adequately addressed through specialty mental health referrals. Oftentimes, the lack of communication between mental health clinicians and PCPs created frustration and confusion.

IPC is more than simply placing BHPs in PC settings. It is a practice transformation approach, and a strong investment in whole person care is its foundation. At its core it relies heavily on the biopsychosocial approach. While most physicians agree with the biopsychosocial model in theory, implementation is quite complex, and it is unlikely that any one clinician can address every need of a patient. Most medical settings are very fast paced, and the number of patients seen can be quite high. Even when multiple clinicians are involved in a patient's care, there are often factors that are overlooked or unable to be addressed.

The IPC model is based on the idea of a *patient-centered medical home* (PCMH), initially created by pediatricians, and later adopted by the other PC professions. The goal is for the patient and their PCP(s) to develop a relationship that results in positive health care outcomes because the setting allows most of the needs of the patient to be met on-site, and the PCP can refer off-site when specialty services are needed. The PCMH recognizes that PC involves a population-based model based on tenants that underscore safety and quality; a whole-person orientation; patients having a personal physician; coordinated and integrated care; enhanced access; and payment for added value. Originally, PCMHs were described as consisting of physician-led treatment teams, but as the concept evolved, it became clear that the treatment teams within a PCMH can be led by whatever health care provider is most appropriate in that role, regardless of discipline (e.g., a clinical health psychologist might lead a team focused on identifying patients with depressive disorders and offering them a variety of treatment options that would include pharmacological treatments offered by a physician consulting with a pharmacist). Patient encounters in an IPC setting by a BHP are generally more problem focused and briefer than those in specialty mental health visits.

PCMH refers to patients having a medical home that is patient-centered with multiple layers

Patient-Centered Medical Home (PCMH) Tenets

Personal Primary Care Provider

Patients have an identified PCP for first point of contact, as well as for longitudinal and comprehensive care.

Safety and Quality

Evidence-based methods integrate the latest technology, decision support tools, and registries, and the PCMH continually emphasizes quality improvement.

Whole-Person Orientation

The PCMH addresses acute, chronic, preventive, and end-of-life care, and addresses both physical and mental health.

Physician-Directed Medical Practice

Physicians tend to be the leads in PC settings, but some activities are led by other health care providers as appropriate.

Coordinated and Integrated Care

A PCP facilitates referrals and access to resources.

Enhanced Access

Easy availability of appointments and resources for patients as well access to communication with health care team.

Payment for Added Value

Payment structures reflect the importance of PCMHs.

A warm handoff is a transfer of care between two health care providers in real time

Various IPC settings operate differently, but typically maintain common processes such as warm handoffs, team-based care, and integration of patient collaboration. In settings with IPC, if a medical provider identifies a behavioral health need, the PCP would introduce the BHP to the patient. In other words, the patient is being seen by the BHP during the actual appointment originally scheduled solely with the PCP after the PCP has met with the patient and identified a need for BHP involvement. The BHP would assess and treat the patient's behavioral concerns and then consult back with the PCP. For example, a warm handoff might occur when a PCP identifies that a patient has suicidal ideation, and the PCP wants a more thorough assessment of the patient's status and a safety plan. For an example of a safety plan, see Appendix 1. Warm handoffs also center around less life-threatening concerns such as sleep problems, recent trauma, grief, panic attacks, and nonadherence to medical regimens. More details about warm handoffs will be provided in the treatment section of this book (see Section 4.1 Methods of Treatment). Additionally, at times, a PCP and a BHP may pre-plan to have a joint visit with a patient. This optimizes care coordination and best use of the patient's time, because the patient does not have to attend two visits. However, at times scheduling issues or other factors can create barriers (Gass et al., 2023).

There is strong evidence supporting the effectiveness of IPC (Archer et al., 2012; Nederveld et al., 2023; Reiss-Brennan et al., 2016; Schmidt et al., 2018). Research shows that IPC increases access to care for patients; leads to equivalent or better clinical outcomes than treatment as usual; increases patient involvement regarding their own self-care plan; and decreases health care expenditures.

The success of IPC within any given clinical operation should be based on solid clinical outcomes, operational consistency and reliability, and financial viability. Additionally, studies show that PCPs report higher job satisfaction and sense of efficacy in IPC settings versus nonintegrated settings. The evidence supporting the treatment of anxiety and depression through IPC is especially strong. Patients also report feeling less stigma receiving mental health services in a PC setting as opposed to in traditional mental health settings (Bluestein & Cubic, 2009; Hunter et al., 2024; Lang, 2005).

Bidirectional IPC refers to the integration of PCPs into specialty mental health settings

Given the success of IPC, bidirectional IPC has gained traction over the last decade to attempt to address the reality that individuals with serious mental illness often develop serious health conditions and die at significantly earlier ages than their peers, most likely because they have not accessed medical care. In contrast to IPC, this approach largely caters to individuals with serious mental illness. The goal of the approach is to make the medical care easily accessible, so that patients with serious mental illness do not need to navigate the complexities of the health care system. The evidence for bidirectional IPC is growing (Mauer & Jarvis, 2010).

The *Triple Aim Initiative* launched in 2008 by the Institute for Healthcare Improvement contributed significantly to the popularity of IPC models (Berwick et al., 2008). This initiative underscored the importance of health care systems focusing on improving patient experience and outcome and overall patient population health, while decreasing per capita health care costs. In 2014, this initiative was expanded to focus on the *quadruple aim*, which adds a focus on health care provider well-being given the high rate of burnout in health care disciplines (Bodenheimer & Sinsky, 2014).

Ultimately the goal of IPC is to ensure that all patients receive what they need, no matter how they engage with the medical system. In other words, no matter how a patient enters into the health care system, the providers they need will be there to provide the care they need. The language used to describe the integration of clinical behavioral approaches in PC has been diverse and has contributed to confusion and difficulty researching many of the concepts embedded in IPC. In 2013, C. J. Peek and colleagues worked with the Agency for Health Care Research and Quality to try to define integrated care concepts to be able to allow for more effective practice-level outcome research (Peek & National Integration Academy Council, 2013). The Substance Abuse and Mental Health Services Administration (SAMSHA) has also created definitions that help link different models to behavioral and structural anchors (Hoge et al., 2014).

Despite efforts to standardize some of the models in IPC, there is still considerable variability. When using the term "IPC," some authors are referring to a colocated practice that is offering what would generally be considered as traditional specialty mental health services. Others are referring to a *collaborative care model* (CoCM; see Section 2.2.2 Collaborative Care Model), while still others are referring to the *primary care behavioral health* (PCBH) model (see Section 2.2.1 Primary Care Behavioral Health). Both models will be described in more detail in Section 2.2 Methods of Care Delivery. When details about how clinics are practicing do emerge, the reality is that most are using hybrid approaches that draw from a variety of models, which have been used for integration.

Another challenge to IPC is a shortage of BHPs who have been trained in IPC settings. Because a unique set of skills and competencies is required, traditionally trained BHPs do not generally fare well in this environment. Education and training efforts have intensified to create a workforce that has the necessary skills, knowledge, and attitudes to function successfully in IPC, but current demand far exceeds the supply.

1.2 Overview

Throughout recent history, individuals have relied on general practitioners to provide the majority of their health care needs. However, after World War II, medical specialties became more prominent, to the point that by the 1960s PC was largely being driven out of existence. In response to this, the fields of family medicine, and later internal medicine and obstetrics and gynecology, started developing departments within academic medicine centers to create more PCPs and PC services (Friedman, 1978). Over time, PC reemerged as a fundamental component of the health care system, but PCPs continue to face challenges in terms of reimbursement for services and a provider shortage. In contrast to providers in specialty health care, PCPs often receive lower compensation and experience higher burnout rates. Accessing PC in rural areas can also be a challenge, and it has been shown that the overall PCP workforce is composed of older providers with limited diversity (Health Resources and Services Administration, 2024), although the general population is becoming increasingly diverse. The anticipated shortage of practicing physicians in PC has also led the way to increased involvement of APPs to address patient concerns, especially in rural areas where the number of health care professionals can often be quite low.

PC settings provide a wide range of health care services to a large and diverse population of patients

The diversity of services provided in PC settings is huge. These health services often include preventive services (e.g., screenings for diabetes, cancer, heart disease), acute services (e.g., cold and flu management), disease diagnosis (e.g., diabetes), management of chronic health conditions (e.g., arthritis), and wellness checkups. While the size of each PCP's panel of patients may vary, the number is typically identified as 2,500 (Murray & Tantau, 2000) but other authors have suggested that this size of a patient panel is not viable (Murray & Tantau, 2000; Raffoul et al., 2016). On average PCPs report seeing approximately 20 patients per clinic-day. While some care delivered is about maintaining wellness, in general, the setting is fast-paced, and complex medical and behavioral presentations are regularly addressed. Providers need to be flexible and comfortable with diverse patients with diverse needs. BHPs are valued by PCPs because they can expand the PCPs' ability to address the behavioral health needs of their patients (e.g., depression, anxiety, trauma) in more depth and allow the provider to move onto seeing other patients to keep the workflow advancing (Bluestein & Cubic, 2009; Hunter et al., 2024; Mitchell, Olson, & Randolph, 2022).

PCPs understand the value of the *biopsychosocial model* – that is, a recognition of the bidirectional influences biological, psychological, and social factors have on health status. By incorporating this understanding of the domains related to genetics, physiology, biochemistry, cognition, mood, behavior, and ecological context (e.g., culture, interpersonal relationships, environment, etc.) and how they bidirectionally impact each other, IPC can thrive (Bluestein & Cubic, 2009). Consequently, most PC practices aspire to have IPC, if possible. In an IPC model there is no wrong door for the patient to enter into the health care system. Regardless of the manner of entry for health care, the patients have all of their medical and behavioral health needs met.

Therefore, a practice shifting toward IPC should build on the existing clinical processes in place, while shifting the practice's culture in a way that allows embracing of IPC. As the field of PC has transitioned conceptually to a goal of IPC, many practices still lack a BHP or enough BHPs to successfully offer services to patients (Rameez & Nasir, 2023). Given that many BHPs are also trained to provide services in specialty mental health, IPC continues to be a goal, but one that is not necessarily achievable in some areas, especially rural areas throughout the United States. For practices invested in IPC, convincing a practice to shift to IPC involves underscoring how the model is patient centered, empirically based, and allows for solid team-based care (Beehler et al., 2024; Bluestein & Cubic, 2009; Fraser et al., 2018; Koehler et al., 2020). Involvement of all parties regarding how the workflow should be redesigned, and how to assure quality improvement occurs, will increase buy-in to IPC.

It is important that BHPs who work in the setting be able to triage patient needs quickly to avoid backing up the clinic. Ideally, the PCP will be able to succinctly discuss with the BHP the patient and their needs prior to a warm handoff, and the BHP will be able to do a quick medical chart review, especially focusing on the synopsis of the patient's medical issues, medications, and sociocultural data. However, on many occasions, the BHP will be interacting with a patient with limited advanced information and will need to do a cursory case conceptualization and preliminary diagnostic formulation to be able to offer a brief intervention or recommendation for a course of action if a more extensive intervention is needed. Documentation of a warm handoff is generally embedded in the note for the PCP visit and should only include key points from the encounter. The bottom line is that IPC requires a willingness to alter planned activities as needed.

BHPs in IPC need to recognize that the pace of care in IPC is quick, with encounters typically lasting 7–20 minutes

For true IPC to occur, all participants in a PC practice must participate in supporting the concept. This includes leadership, PCPs, nurses, ancillary providers (e.g., pharmacists), BHPs, staff, and most importantly, patients. Additionally, within PC, BHPs must be able to create a balance between scheduled appointments for brief psychotherapy, and availability for warm handoffs and other lengthier consultations. It is also important that patients are informed about what IPC looks like and how information is shared. Similarities to and differences from specialty mental health need to be described to the patient as well. It is not uncommon for a BHP in an IPC setting to be in the middle of a meeting, supervision of another health care provider, or a patient encounter, when they are asked to do a warm handoff. In this circumstance, the BHP needs to evaluate the seriousness of the issues the warm handoff will address and balance that against the ongoing activity they are participating in, to determine which takes precedence. This is just one way that the IPC setting requires flexibility and a comfort zone in dealing with the unpredictable.

1.3 Competencies Needed

IPC requires practitioners with a unique set of competencies. BHPs who have completed practicums, internships, and/or fellowships in IPC settings during their training are ideal for working in IPC. However, traditionally trained BHPs can adapt to IPC settings with substantial training. The setting requires flexibility, the ability to think quickly on your feet, a willingness to work with a diverse number of presenting problems, and interpersonal skills that allow collegial and effective communication with colleagues from other disciplines. Warm handoffs, the transferring of care from a medical provider to a BHP in the presence of the patient and family, are common, and as stated earlier, rarely does a BHP have much information about the patient prior to the encounter, and they will often have limited time to assess the patient and create a useful treatment plan to convey to the patient's provider.

Multiple sets of competencies underscore the knowledge, skills, and attitudes needed for IPC settings

In 2013, Nash et al. published the essential competencies for psychologists in PCMHs (Nash et al., 2013). Most importantly, this document introduced the PC ethic, a guiding principle resulting in an appreciation, openness, and willingness to engage in interprofessional PC environments. This document was followed in 2014 by a publication by the Interorganizational Work Group for the American Psychological Association, that listed the competencies needed for psychology in PC (McDaniel et al., 2014). These competencies centered around the clusters of science, systems, professionalism, relationships, application, and education. For each cluster, essential components and samples of behavioral anchors were illustrated. Case vignettes were also provided. This article underscored the importance of BHPs being trained in team-based care, population-based health care, and brief assessment and intervention methods. That same year, SAMSHA published its "Core Competencies for Integrated Behavioral Health and Primary Care" (Hoge et al., 2014). This document's goal was to provide PC settings with a resource that would allow them to determine what characteristics BHPs would need to thrive in those settings, and to create competencies that transcended disciplines within the field of behavioral health, which would position any type of BHP for successful integration. The competencies focused on the areas of interpersonal communication, collaboration and teamwork, screening and assessment, care planning and care coordination, intervention, cultural competence and adaption, systems-oriented practice, practice-based learning and quality improvement, and informatics.

In 2009, a collaboration called Interprofessional Education Collaborative (IPEC), with representatives from dentistry, nursing, medicine, osteopathic medicine, pharmacy, and public health, created core competencies for interprofessional collaborative practice. These were updated in 2016 and again in 2023 (Interprofessional Education Collaborative [IPEC], 2023). The goal of these competencies was to move from profession-specific competencies to competencies that transcend each profession and focus on the knowledge, skills, and attitudes needed for interprofessional collaboration. A fundamental recommendation of the IPEC was interdisciplinary educational opportunities to achieve the competencies needed to successfully provide team-based care.

The cross-cutting theme across all of these defined competencies discussed in this book is the importance of having specialty-based expertise offered through team-based care in a PC setting. When individuals understand the role of others, as well as their own role, in providing patient care, the quality of care is improved, and patient satisfaction increases. Provider satisfaction is higher as well, especially in rural areas (English et al., 2024).

Engaging in a team-based approach can lead to enhanced well-being among health care providers, who no longer feel like they are solely responsible for every aspect of a patient's care, because they have team members who can assist them (Gunn, 2024).

1.4 Context Matters

Some settings will benefit from a model that incorporates a BHP into specialty subclinics (e.g. an intensive interdisciplinary diabetes clinic), whereas others may best be served by having the BHP available during clinic hours for warm handoffs only, while another might benefit from colocated clinics (e.g., on-site brief therapy) intermingled with warm handoffs for acute concerns (e.g., a patient expressing suicidal ideation). IPEC works most effectively when a needs assessment has been conducted and the model of care has been adapted to meet the needs of the patient population being treated and the providers involved in that treatment. During the assessment, a multitude of factors are considered, including patient characteristics, provider characteristics, resources available, and institutional strengths and barriers, among other factors. Data are gathered from the individuals who will be impacted by a shift to IPC. Patients, their families, and providers should all be surveyed, or interviewed (if possible), to obtain their perspectives regarding unmet behavioral health concerns in a typical PC model and ways that integration of a BHP could improve the overall physical and mental health of patients receiving services at the clinic. Best strategies for integrating a BHP should also be discussed. The needs assessment will also be able to rely on a number of data sources (e.g., reports regarding number and type of visits, presenting concerns, procedures performed over the course of a year) to create a care model that best utilizes BHPs.

IPC looks very different across very different health care settings

A needs assessment is used to assess the gaps within a setting that limit the system's ability to provide optimal care

The needs assessment takes into account characteristics of the patient population (e.g., age ranges, health statuses, races, disability statuses, genders, socioeconomic statuses, and languages spoken) because the services needed in downtown Chicago will likely be very different from those needed in rural West Virginia. For example, BHPs working in rural West Virginia will rarely utilize interpretative services, because the language spoken is generally English, but in New York City, interpretative services may be a routine component of the visits a BHP provides in PC. The needs assessment should be the driving factor for determining how much of a BHP's time is focused on warm handoffs, brief assessments and therapy, participation in interdisciplinary clinics, and consultations. Age ranges become a highly significant factor in the needs assessment for IPC, because the skills needed to work with children, adolescents, adults, and geriatric patients vary considerably.

Providers also need to strike a balance between diagnostic assessments and follow-up appointments, if therapy is offered within the PC location, because once they have started therapy with a patient, it is imperative that they are available to that patient until their treatment is completed or transferred to a specialized mental health clinician.

It is also important to note that a needs assessment should be an ongoing process. The needs of clinics and their patient populations are always evolving. Successful IPC practices continually reassess their services to determine ways to improve the quality of services provided. To assist providers in evaluating their potential for creating a mode of IPC that will likely be successful, providers can utilize the Behavioral Health Integration Capacity

Assessment tool (https://www.cms.gov/files/zip/ricresource-behavioral healthintegrationcapacityassessment.zip).This tool was created by Resources for Integrated Care and provides questions and interactive scoring for a provider to assess their clinic's readiness for IPC. A guide for the instrument is also included on the website to provide details about how the tool was created and should be completed. Categories measured include understanding your entity's population, assessing the entity's infrastructure, determining the existing culture for support, evaluating screening processes in place and ability to identify high-risk populations, assessing optimal integration, and reviewing financing factors. Responses across these categories are summarized to determine the entity's readiness for integration of behavioral health and PC. Recommendations are made regarding the potential for colocated versus embedded IPC.

One of the most important characteristics of IPC involves BHPs being flexible and adaptable. Although the differences in setting may be starker when comparing pediatric with adult with geriatric settings, there are still substantial differences within each of these. The needs of a PC practice that provides educational offerings may be significantly different from the needs of one that focuses solely on clinical care delivery. This underscores the importance of the needs assessment. In addition to tools already discussed, there are multiple publicly available measures for a practice to use to determine its readiness for IPC. They include the Atlas of Integrated Behavioral Healthcare Quality Measures (Agency for Healthcare Research and Quality, 2013), the Behavioral Health Integration Capacity Assessment tool (U.S. Centers for Medicare & Medical Services, 2024), the Practice Integration Profile – Revised (Rose et al., 2023), and the Readiness for Integration Care Questionnaire (Scott et al., 2017), to name but a few.

2

Theories and Models

2.1 Continuum of Care

While many settings describe themselves as integrated, the level of integration varies greatly across sites. On one end of the continuum would be a complete lack of integration where medical providers and BHPs operate in silos with limited or no communication regarding patient care. On the opposite end of the spectrum would be a clinic staffed with medical providers and BHPs who work side by side daily, offering individual health care and programs to patients and their families.

There is a continuum of integration, but the goal of IPC is population-based health care delivery, and a framework for operating in IPC settings is needed. In 2006, Barbara Mauer and colleagues, through the National Council for Community Behavioral Healthcare, conceptualized that a *four-quadrant model* could allow for health care settings to adequately triage patients effectively to meet their needs (Mauer, 2006) (Figure 1). The guiding principles from this model can help PC clinics to determine how much of the patient care that will be provided should be delivered by the PCP, BHP, or other team members. The model divides the patient population into four groups, while acknowledging that over time, individuals may move from quadrant to quadrant depending on their health care needs. *Quadrant 1* comprises individuals with both low physical and behavioral health care needs, and with this subgroup, health care providers focus on maintaining wellness and screening for high-risk conditions, such as anxiety and depression. *Quadrant II* consists of individuals with low physical health needs but high behavioral health needs. Bidirectional IPC might be best indicated for this subgroup given the likely high involvement of BHPs in their care. *Quadrant III* reflects individuals with high physical health complexity and low behavioral health needs. PCPs will have the primary role with this subgroup of patients, providing care and referrals to specialists as needed. BHPs will concentrate on providing care centered on coping with medical concerns, adherence to medical regimens, and improving lifestyle factors that can compromise health (e.g., sleep, exercise, nutrition, stress). *Quadrant IV* is made up of individuals with both high physical and behavioral health complexity and risk. The entire team of health care providers in IPC may be involved in their care, as well as many specialists outside of the PC. Care for this subgroup requires the highest level of care coordination, communication, and documentation; and utilizes the most resources. Medical insurance companies are very cognizant of the fact that

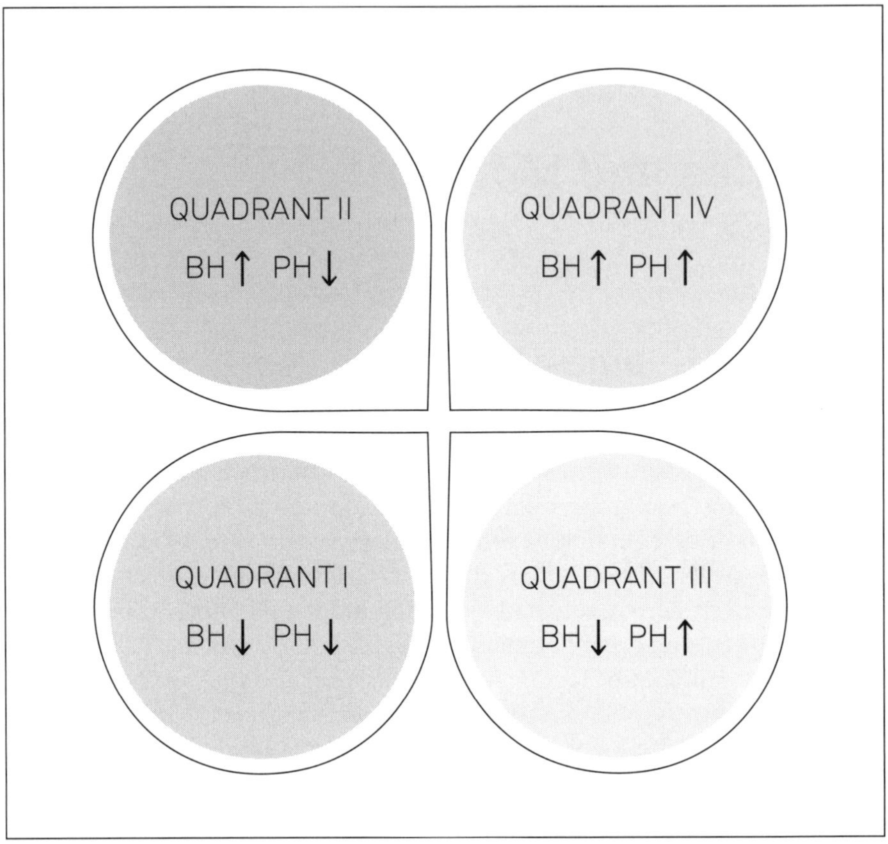

Figure 1. Four-quadrant model: behavioral or physical health continuum for risk or complexity (low to high). BH = behavioral health needs; PH = physical health needs. Based on Mauer, 2006.

this group is their most expensive source of obligations, and promoting IPC for this group can be beneficial for insurers.

2.2 Methods of Care Delivery

Numerous health care models that integrate medical and behavioral treatments have been implemented in PC settings

The degree of integration between BHPs and PC physicians varies. The nomenclature used includes collaborative, coordinated, colocated, care management, primary care–mental health integration, and blended – among others. Below we will discuss three major models of IPC that have been utilized regularly with strong empirical support. These models are the PCBH (Primary Care Behavioral Health), the CoCM (Collaborative Care Model), and Primary Care–Mental Health Integration (PC-MHI). PCBH is designed to provide patients care when they are dealing with episodic stressors, challenges adhering to health behavior regimens, and with mild to moderate mental health and substance abuse issues. CoCM is a psychiatric monitoring model for more severe mental illnesses or for those who have not responded to PCBH. PC-MHI integrates best aspects of both models.

2.2.1 Primary Care Behavioral Health

PCBH is considered a generalist model that embeds a BHP within a PC practice to provide warm handoffs, assessments, consultations, and brief interventions

In the PCBH model, the BHP does not limit their health care service delivery to only mental health and substance abuse issues; instead, they often treat common health conditions such as pain, obesity, and insomnia. All services provided are evidence-based, and close coordination with the PCP is a necessity. Patients do not begin and end a course of treatment, rather they come in and out of treatment as needed for whatever number of sessions is required. Oftentimes the PCBH provider may only see the patient for one session following a warm handoff. When additional sessions do occur, most often six to eight sessions are considered normative at any given time.

As a result, PCBH attempts to be simultaneously integrated, collaborative, and colocated. Some clinics using a PCBH model are largely integrated, with limited time for colocated therapy sessions, whereas others are largely colocated, with limited time for integrated care. The time allocated to colocation and integration will generally be determined by the number of BHPs within a practice or the needs of a practice. For example, if a PC practice struggles to be able to refer to specialty mental health providers because of a lack of access, the practice may rely more on their BHPs for colocated services than would a practice that has ready access to specialty mental health and, therefore, can utilize their BHPs more for integrated care.

An advantage of the PCBH model is that it can lead to the early identification of factors contributing to chronic diseases and possibly mitigate those factors through interventions such as motivational interviewing and cognitive behavioral techniques (to be discussed in Chapter 4: Treatment). The model has also been shown to improve access to behavioral health services, relationships between providers and their patients, and satisfaction with the health care system, for both patients and their providers (Koehler et al., 2020).

The diversity of the clinical activities that PCBH providers engage in has made it challenging to find empirical evidence for its effectiveness. Therefore, the research behind PCBH that does exist is still advancing, but it is noteworthy that it is already solid. Hunter and colleagues (2018) have provided a qualitative review of published research on PCBH, supporting the utility of the model in terms of increasing patient access to providers, patient satisfaction, provider satisfaction, and positive clinical outcomes.

2.2.2 Collaborative Care Model (CoCM)

The CoCM model focuses on chronic mental health concerns

In contrast to the PCBH model, the CoCM is focused primarily on mental health concerns, most notably those that are chronic, such as persistent depression, severe anxiety disorders, bipolar disorder, schizophrenia, and other serious mental health disorders. The CoCM would also be appropriate for patients who have not been responding to the brief assessments and interventions offered through the PCBH model. A CoCM practice consists of a team that includes the PCP, a psychiatrist, and a case manager. The psychiatrist serves as a consultant to the PCP, and the case manager monitors the patients on a regular basis. When patients are in need of specialty mental health care (i.e., therapy, residential care, inpatient hospitalization) and willing to pursue it, additional clinicians are brought into the treatment team, and the case manager tries to coordinate care with them as well. Patients may be seen over the course of several months, with the case manager generally checking in at least weekly, and with the patient and the team meeting regularly to discuss the patient's progress.

The CoCM has four necessary components to create quality and effectiveness (American Psychiatric Association and Academy of Psychosomatic Medicine, 2016). It is *team-driven*, *population-focused*, *measurement-guided*, and *evidence-based*. When these components are present, the care that patients receive for their mental health concerns in PC is enhanced. Most patients seen in a CoCM practice are cared for within the model, for approximately 6–12 months.

The CoCM relies on registries – that is, databases on patients with certain diagnosed conditions, to track and monitor patients and to identify patients that might benefit from services by a PCP, psychiatrist, and case manager. These registries become data points regarding the success, or lack thereof, regarding an attempted intervention. The research behind the CoCM is strong. Over 80 randomized controlled trials (RCTs) have documented the efficacy of CoCM as an evidence-based method for addressing serious mental health issues within primary care settings (AIMS Center, 2024). Additionally, the CoCM has been shown to be more cost-effective than treatment as usual (AIMS Center, 2024).

2.2.3 Primary Care–Mental Health Integration

PC-MHI is the model of IPC that combines care management and integrated services

The PC-MHI model has frequently been referred to as a blended model that capitalizes on the benefits of the PCBH model and the CoCM by blending them together. This blended model has been utilized by the Veterans Health Administration (VHA), Department of Defense, and large health care systems, such as Cherokee Health Systems and Intermountain Health Systems, with significant effectiveness, as both PCBH (Reiter et al., 2018) and the CoCM (Reist et al., 2022) have strong empirical support. In the VHA, BHPs are placed in PC clinics and work in conjunction with the patients' *patient aligned care team* (PACT) to address patients' mental health needs. The VHA has also created a Center for Integrated Healthcare which gives providers a compendium of resources across a spectrum of types, topics, and levels of expertise (see https://www.mirecc.va.gov/cih-visn2/). The Center for Integrated Healthcare also provides numerous other resources for providers and patients regarding IPC.

The primary challenge regarding implementing PC-MHI in small PC clinics is that many practices, especially those in rural areas, do not have the behavioral health resources found in the VHA. Therefore, it is common for smaller clinics to participate either in a PCBH model or a CoCM, if they are able to have behavioral health clinicians at all.

2.3 Sharing of Information

Confidentiality is considered an inviolable agreement between a patient and a BHP, with only a few exceptions (i.e., suicide risk, abuse of an individual who cannot protect themselves, certain legal scenarios). It is considered unethical for a BHP to release information a patient has shared, except when an exception applies, unless a patient has signed a *release of information* (ROI). Consequently, unless a specialty mental health clinic makes it a practice for patients to release information to their PCPs, a patient rarely initiates the exchange of information. Therefore, one of the most frequent complaints of PCPs is that when they refer a patient to a mental health specialist, they receive little or no feedback about the patient care provided. This puts the PCP in the difficult position of being responsible for the patient's health care outcomes, with no input to, or from, the mental health specialist. It is critical that referring PCPs get timely, responsive, and useful feedback after making a referral to a BHP.

Sharing information related to patient care is a fundamental principle of interprofessional collaboration

Sharing of information about patient care is a basic tenant of interprofessional collaboration (IPC). Patients are informed at the onset of care that the clinic uses a team-based model and that providers will be sharing information to coordinate care and provide the patient with the best possible outcome. Ideally, this is conveyed in the consent form signed by the patient, but also reiterated verbally at the onset of an interaction, which allows the patient to ask questions or express any concerns they might have. Most patients appreciate that their PCP will be kept abreast of any behavioral health assessments or interventions that will be provided, and that their BHP will be apprised of any important health care concerns.

2.4 Documentation

Most training programs in behavioral health fields focus extensively on writing diagnostic assessments, therapy notes, and psychological evaluations that are very detailed. This type of documentation does not work effectively in IPC settings. PCPs have very limited time to review the documentation provided to them by specialists and want *key findings*, especially those that impact or enhance their treatment plan. When possible, succinct verbal feedback is ideal. However, many times the PCP has moved on to other patient encounters and may not be easily accessible. Therefore, in IPC, BHPs are generally encouraged to write succinct notes that highlight the most relevant details that the PCP needs to know. This can be done in several ways. *Subjective, objective, assessment, plan* (SOAP) notes are widely used, but some providers opt to write an *assessment, plan, subjective, objective* (APSO) note to highlight their conclusions quickly for the PCPs in their practice, as the assessment and plan sections are first. Another way to accomplish this is to highlight, or render in bold or red font, the most important messages in the note. Messages should be sent to the PCPs through the electronic health record when an assessment has been completed, a preliminary diagnosis is changed or solidified, or important concerns have been raised by a patient. Details about the intervention recommended also should be conveyed to the PCP so that the PCP can reinforce to the patient what the BHP has recommended.

2.5 Ethical Considerations

Different professions have different ethical guidelines

As in all types of health care delivery, ethical considerations are important in IPC. However, this may be especially challenging in IPC settings because ethical guidance is generally specific to the guild of each discipline, which can create confusion in IPC because of the various disciplines involved. For example, the ethical code of conduct for physicians issued by the American Medical Association allows for colleagues to treat colleagues, while trying to remain sensitive to the potential for ethical conflicts (American Medical Association, 2017). In contrast, the ethical code of conduct for psychologists, issued by the American Psychological Association (2017), and for social workers, issued by the National Association of Social Workers (2021), discourages involvement in dual relationships. Therefore, it is not uncommon for a physician to potentially provide medical care to their behavioral health colleagues, but when reciprocation is expected, the behavioral health clinician would need to avoid providing care to the physician or their family. This can cause confusion and tension within a treatment team.

To date there is no ethical code of conduct that applies across disciplines for IPC settings. Until a cross-cutting ethical code of conduct is developed, both the PCP and BHP have to remain true to their own ethical code of conduct, while working as a team for the overall good of patients. Any conflicts resulting will need to be resolved through expert opinion and collegiality.

Despite the differences, there are areas where all disciplines agree ethically. For example, all disciplines are required to ensure that patient safety is paramount and that no harm is done. All disciplines have an obligation to maintain confidentiality, which is further reinforced by the Health Insurance Portability and Accountability Act (HIPAA). Health care providers also need to be aware of ethical considerations when working with older adults, specifically the need to balance the autonomy of the patient with the desire to protect the patient from harm. This dilemma may arise when dealing with issues of capacity and surrogate decision making (American Psychological Association, 2012). In addition, as mandated reporters, the PCP must also be alert to possible elder abuse or neglect.

3

Assessment and Treatment Indications

3.1 Common Presenting Problems

In addition to the identification of patients with behavioral health needs during their medical appointments, systematic screening processes for behavioral health issues should be implemented in IPC settings. At a minimum, it is important that the screening process be used to evaluate both obvious and more subtle presentations of behavioral health problems.

3.1.1 Children

Pediatric PC settings are often tasked with managing most behavioral health issues presenting in children and adolescents. Families trust their pediatrician to provide them with psychoeducation, counseling, and psychotropic medications (if indicated), and pediatricians report that behavioral health concerns represent a significant portion of the presenting problems they treat (Chien et al., 2022). In fact, some surveys have shown that behavioral health concerns are more prominent than any other issues, especially in adolescents (Centers for Disease Control, 2024). Studies have also shown that visits to the pediatrician focused on behavioral health issues last longer than those scheduled for other health concerns (Gotlieb et al., 2014). Despite the frequency with which pediatricians must address behavioral health issues, many indicate that they are uncomfortable in these situations, especially when prescribing psychotropic medications. However, when a pediatrician wants to refer a child or adolescent to a specialty mental health provider, the patient's family rarely follows through. Additionally, there is a national shortage of child psychiatrists in the United States. It just makes sense that IPC could improve the health care children and adolescents receive.

As in all IPC settings, the behavioral issues that present vary; however, some issues commonly occur in pediatric settings. In pediatric IPC, common issues treated by a BHP include distress related to medical procedures (e.g., vaccinations, pap smear, stiches), difficulty taking pills, lack of adherence to medical regimens, disruptive behavior, anxiety, depression, bullying, eating disorders, poor sleep, challenges with toileting, obesity, and chronic pain. Preliminary evaluations and treatments for attention-deficit/hyperactivity disorder (ADHD), autism spectrum disorder, and other developmental disorders may also be conducted. Additionally, a significant amount of time is often used to teach parenting skills. See section on parent-child interaction therapy (PCIT) in Section 4.1.1 Interventions.

3.1.2 Adults

There is a myriad of ways that BHPs can help in PC clinics treating primarily adults. Leveraging a BHP as a consultant and a team member in PC can improve the quality of care that the PCP is able to provide. Most notably, depression and anxiety are common presentations in which a PCP will appreciate the insights of a BHP. Research shows that PCPs diagnose depression and anxiety disorders most frequently and write considerably more antidepressant prescriptions than specialty mental health providers (Lester et al., 2023). Patients often discuss these mental health conditions at their medical visit because of the close relationship they have developed with their PCP, and find it more convenient to get all of their physical and mental health care in one setting.

The motivational interviewing skills that BHPs bring to a health care setting can inspire a patient to work toward abstinence from alcohol or other drug abuse as well as to make health behavior changes to manage chronic conditions such as high blood pressure (see the subsection Motivational Interviewing, in Section 4.1.1 Interventions).

A significant number of warm handoffs that happen in an adult IPC setting may be related to issues of risk. PC settings are recommended to have protocols for how to address patients who are suicidal or homicidal, and these protocols should include the involvement of a BHP when one is available. A BHP can spend more time with the patient evaluating their suicidal ideation, intent, plan, and reasons for not acting on their plan. The BHP is also likely to be better informed about resources for the patient, whether those be inpatient or outpatient, and how to ensure that the patient is able to access those resources. As a team, a BHP and PCP can ensure the patient's safety, and demonstrate care and compassion while doing so by completing a safety plan (see Appendix 1).

Adult settings may also offer interdisciplinary clinics for patients with certain conditions (e.g., obesity, diabetes, or chronic obstructive pulmonary disease), and clinics often welcome the inclusion of BHPs because of their specialized level of expertise in changing behaviors.

3.1.3 Older Adults

Older adults (age 65 years and over) in the United States are now accounting for a higher proportion of the patients seen in PC populations (Huffstetler & Topmiller, 2024). This increasingly aging population utilizes the health care system at a high frequency, because multiple comorbid conditions and chronic health conditions are common, also resulting in more complex medical visits. Therefore, PCPs must be knowledgeable about the needs of their older adult patients to treat their unique concerns and efficiently manage their care, including their mental health needs. Subsequently, in IPC settings, BHPs also must be prepared to address the unique needs of geriatric populations. In doing so, all health care professionals must avoid both obvious and subtle ageism – that is, prejudice, stereotyping, and discrimination against older adults – as it is associated with numerous adverse health outcomes for older adults. These negative outcomes include poorer cognitive performance, less functional health, lower well-being, and earlier mortality (Levy et al., 2012). Bryant et al. (2012) also found that negative self-perceptions of aging can contribute to poor mental health. Changes to vision, hearing, physical mobility, and cognition, secondary to age, also need to be taken into consideration. For example, providers may need to change the volume and rate of their speech, use larger print visuals (e.g., for self-report scales), and have better awareness of environmental factors such as lighting or background noise in examination and therapy rooms for geriatric patients. Polypharmacy issues must also be addressed. Polypharmacy refers to situations where multiple drugs are being used to treat a medical condition(s) and, unfortunately, in geriatric patients this is often the case. The use of multiple drugs increases the risk of adverse reactions because of the interplay between medications.

It is also important to recognize that older adults are also more likely to feel stigmatized if they seek mental health and are thus more likely to seek mental health care in PC settings (Elshaikh et al., 2023). BHPs can provide brief treatment in PC settings for mood stabilization, adjustment and grief issues, cognitive strategies to manage memory loss, anxiety, trauma, and other issues. It is also important to consider the family system for older adults, as family members often accompany older adult patients to their PCP appointments, serve as caregivers, provide collateral information, and/or help with follow-through on treatment recommendations (Molinari, 2011).

Older adults are more likely to be sensitive to stigma associated with mental health treatment

Cognitive impairment may also be present in geriatric patients. IPC providers must be able to recognize healthy aging, and differentiate it from cognitive deterioration. Luckily, PC settings are a perfect environment for recognizing changes, as geriatric patients typically trust their PCPs and see them frequently. BHPs can further assist a PCP in determining if cognitive decline is occurring, by administering a mental status examination (MSE; Sultzer, 1994), Montreal Cognitive Assessment (MoCA; Nasreddine et al., 2005), Cognistat (Kiernan et al., 1995), or Repeatable Battery for the Assessment of Neuropsychological Status (RBANS; Randolph et al., 1998), which are fairly quick assessments to administer in a PC setting and can provide a baseline and serial assessments.

3.2 Universal Screenings Versus Targeted Populations

The rule of thumb in medicine is that you do not screen for anything if you cannot effectively treat the disorder or provide appropriate referrals or

Screening is done when the disorder can be effectively treated or managed with appropriate referrals or resources

resources. Therefore, PC clinics are tasked with ensuring that they are prepared to address any physical or mental health concerns that are identified. The clinics also need to make sure that they have clear processes in place for how patients are triaged once identified as having a behavioral health concern, and that those processes are widely known, not only by all PCPs, but by nursing and other staff as well. Most PC practices feel confident in screening for common medical concerns (e.g., diabetes, hypertension, etc.), common substance use and misuse (e.g., tobacco, alcohol), and common behavioral health concerns (e.g., depressive and anxiety disorders). However, clinic staff may be less comfortable with screening for behavioral health concerns such as eating disorders, trauma, and more specific substance use disorders (e.g., use of opioids, crystal methamphetamine).

Universal screenings are now recommended for depression and anxiety in PC clinics, and the Patient Health Questionnaire–9 (PHQ-9; Kroenke et al., 2001) and Generalized Anxiety Disorder–7 (GAD-7; Spitzer et al., 2006) are commonly used with adults in PC settings. For pediatric populations, the Children's Depression Inventory (CDI; Kovacs, 1985) for children under age 12, or Patient Health Questionnaire (PHQ-A; Johnson et al., 2002) for adolescents will commonly be used. For geriatric populations, the Geriatric Depression Scale (GDS; Scogin et al., 2000) may be used instead of the PHQ-9, but the PHQ-9 is still most commonly used. Cognitive screening is also recommended as a universal screening during adult wellness visits for geriatric patients. Most often the MSE (Sultzer, 1994) and MoCA (Nasreddine et al., 2005) are used. However, when indicated, measures such as the RBANS (Randolph et al., 1998) or Cognistat (Kiernan et al., 1995) can be used.

Each clinic will need to determine if they have the capacity to screen for more behavioral health conditions other than depression and anxiety, and have BHPs and other resources when other problems are present. Clinics also need to recognize that when screenings are conducted, false negatives do occur. Therefore, clinics should have a plan for how to address patients who appear to have a mental health concern but in fact may have other needs that must be addressed first (e.g., social determinants of health).

3.3 The 5As Model

The *5As model*, most notably advocated for by Hunter et al. (2024), consists of five steps based on self-determination theory. Self-determination theory is a framework for understanding human motivation and the factors that impact it, both internal and external (Ryan & Deci, 2000). In essence, the theory focuses on the role that autonomy, competence and relatedness play in whether an individual is motivated for change or not. The five steps of the 5As model are *ask*, *advise*, *assess*, *assist*, and *arrange*. During the *ask* phase, the BHP will focus on discussing the patient's current behavior: both how it is effective for them, and how it is problematic. In the *advise* phase, the clinician and patient identify an agreed-upon point of change. In the *assess* phase, the clinician will utilize motivational interviewing to determine the patient's willingness for change. Goal setting is the primary task for the *assist* phase, and the *arrange* phase is focused on follow-up. Many BHPs are trained to utilize the 5As model to direct their IPC sessions.

3.4 Stepped Care

Stepped care in primary care delivers effective treatment with minimal resources

Stepped care is a model for providing care within PC that focuses on the most effective treatments using the fewest resources. If medical situations can be handled at the PC level, then they are. Specialty care is only utilized when PC cannot sufficiently address the needs of the patient. In other words, a hierarchy of care is used that goes from the least to the most intensive care required. For IPC, this would mean that the PCP would address most behavioral health issues, if possible, then a BHP within IPC would be brought in as needed, and then a referral to specialty mental health care would occur only if required.

3.5 Treat Versus Refer (Serving as a Bridge)

While the diversity of clinical presentations in PC is vast, PC is not the proper place to address all behavioral health issues that patients experience. Conditions that can generally be managed in PC include depressive disorders, anxiety disorders, trauma-related disorders, eating disorders, ADHD, pain, sleep disorders, substance abuse disorders, and somatic disorders, as long as they are mild or moderate in severity. More severe occurrences will be best addressed by specialty mental health services. Psychotic disorders, bipolar disorders, autism, and severe substance abuse disorders, ideally, will not be managed in PC.

Regularly, BHPs in IPC are tasked with making a decision about whether a patient's behavioral health issues can be managed in PC or need to be managed in a specialty mental health setting. However, even though it may be clear that a patient needs more services than can be offered in PC, as many traditional behavioral health settings and providers have long waitlists, and some patients will not agree to seek behavioral health services outside of PC.

Subsequently, IPC BHPs need to create a bridge to more extensive behavioral health care. This bridge may involve more frequent encounters in the IPC setting, longer encounters in the IPC setting, integration of additional resources (e.g., support groups, apps, books), and closer coordination of care with the PCP. For patients reluctant to be seen in specialty mental health settings, the bridge may also include motivational interviewing and psychoeducation to reduce the stigma the patient may fear they will experience if they seek more specific behavioral health treatment.

3.6 Telehealth in IPC

Telehealth is defined as the provision of health care remotely through telecommunication technology. Most commonly telehealth services are provided through telephone contact or a virtual visit on an electronic device. While some telehealth services have been offered for decades, the COVID pandemic catapulted the use of telehealth services to protect the public and health care providers in 2020 from unnecessary exposure to the COVID virus. Since then, telehealth has become a mainstream method for behavioral service delivery. In IPC settings, telehealth can be used for warm handoffs when BHPs are not on site and allows for increased access to point-of-care treatment. Provision of services through telehealth is particularly important in rural areas and for patients who are disadvantaged and may not have the ability to present to the clinic easily (e.g., no transportation, medically incapacitated).

4

Treatment

4.1 Methods of Treatment

BHPs frequently review the schedules of providers for patients who may benefit from a warm handoff

A key feature of IPC is the administration of *warm handoffs*. Warm handoffs refer to brief encounters (approximately 10 to 15 minutes) between BHPs and patients that aim to "bridge" the patient into receiving appropriate behavioral health treatment. PCPs identify patients who are appropriate for a warm handoff during clinic encounters. Having BHPs present in nursing and attending physician areas of a clinic can facilitate warm handoffs because they are able to hear discussions amongst providers that can highlight patients that may be appropriate for a warm handoff. Additionally, BHPs that are present in these clinic areas for a designated period of time (e.g., afternoon from 1:00 p.m. to 5:00 p.m.) can spend time reviewing provider's schedules for appropriate warm handoffs. This process is called scrubbing. Consultation with the referring PCP before a warm handoff gives the BHP a general sense of what concerns may be discussed with a patient and whether the referring provider may want to see the patient again once the warm handoff is completed. It is important for BHPs to be aware of how much time may be used in a clinic room for a warm handoff given the common problem of limited clinic rooms in PC settings. Having a designated room for warm handoffs that require more than 15 minutes (typically the office of a BHP) helps facilitate the workflows of referring providers.

Warm handoffs that are completed by BHPs involve targeted assessments and interventions for a wide range of physical and mental health concerns including depression, anxiety, interpersonal problems (e.g., marital problems), suicide risk, medication adherence, and lifestyle changes such as weight management. Other concerns that may be addressed in a warm handoff include issues related to lack of access to fundamental resources such as housing, air conditioning or heat, winter clothing, or food. Accordingly, BHPs benefit from having knowledge of resources in their clinic and community that can help address these concerns. Furthermore, having clinic policies and procedures for addressing suicidality and homicidal concerns can facilitate warm handoffs in cases in which patients endorse suicidal and/or homicidal ideations, plans, or active intent in the clinic. BHPs are typically involved in numerous activities including individual outpatient care, teaching, or research activities, and thus having a procedure in place to locate BHPs when a warm handoff is deemed appropriate can improve the completion of warm handoffs in a clinic. Patients may also benefit from being referred directly to services in the community that can provide more intensive care such as long-term psychotherapy, and knowing about these resources can facilitate such referrals.

BHPs tend to become more comfortable with warm handoffs the more they complete them

Warm handoffs may be challenging encounters given the lack of time to prepare before seeing a patient. Assessment by the BHP in a warm handoff is focused on addressing the concerns of the referring provider and may involve the use of brief questionnaires for common PC presentations (e.g., anxiety, depression, trauma, substance use). Behavioral health interventions may also be introduced in a warm handoff such as safety planning, deep-breathing exercises, review of behavioral activation principles, grounding techniques, worksheets that provide resources for interventions such as meditation, or suggestions about various apps that might be helpful for the presenting problem. Giving a patient a "tool" to take home after completing a warm handoff often helps them see immediate symptom relief and provides them with an example of the types of interventions they can learn in psychotherapy. Warm handoffs have been shown to increase the likelihood of a patient attending an initial behavioral health appointment and improve patient satisfaction with the treatment they receive in PC (Mitchell et al., 2022).

Warm handoff notes should be brief and concise

Documentation of warm handoffs is typically completed within the medical chart encounter of the referring provider. Notes for warm handoffs are most helpful when they are brief and provide concise recommendations. Providing referring providers with brief in-person feedback and recommendations after a warm handoff is completed can facilitate appropriate treatment of the patient and build rapport with the PCPs. Documentation of the assessment of suicide concerns is especially important and should include justifications for decisions (e.g., reasons a patient was deemed safe to leave the clinic with appropriate follow-up vs. reasons a decision was made to transfer patient to the emergency department).

BHPs may also provide brief psychotherapy to patients in PC. Providing patients with psychotherapy in a PC context has the benefit of reducing the stigma related to receiving mental health treatment. Brief colocated psychotherapy referrals come from PCPs and often follow a warm handoff. They typically involve six to eight sessions (about 30 minutes per session, occurring every 2 to 3 weeks). Short-term psychotherapy in PC begins with an intake session that focuses on the assessment of the patient's presenting concerns, mental health treatment history, family mental health history, current stressors, substance use, relevant life history, and a discussion of goals for therapy. Initial sessions also include assessment of a wide range of mental health problems including depression, anxiety, trauma exposure history, mania, psychosis, disordered eating, substance use, and sleep problems. Patients in PC often present with comorbid physical health problems, and thus an assessment of physical health factors such as chronic conditions (e.g., diabetes, hypertension) should also be completed. Symptom severity, history of presenting concerns, and patient goals inform whether an initial intake session should also involve a discussion of transferring to long-term psychotherapy at the conclusion of brief psychotherapy. If a patient is starting long-term psychotherapy, doing it as soon as possible is the best option. After the completion of the intake session for brief outpatient psychotherapy, BHPs frequently alert the referring PCP (via the medical chart or a brief in-person meeting) with their impression of the patient (e.g., mental health diagnoses, psychosocial factors that are impacting the patient, brief description of treatment plan for subsequent brief outpatient psychotherapy). This communication continues over the course of the brief outpatient psychotherapy and ensures that both the BHP and PCP are working together to meet the needs of patients.

Interventions in brief, colocated, psychotherapy predominantly involve the introduction of *cognitive behavior therapy* (CBT) principles including psychoeducation. Patients are also introduced to interventions such as paced-breathing exercises, progressive muscle relaxation, and meditation; these are skills that patients can practice in their daily life, often with the help of resources such as worksheets and videos or websites that have recordings of these interventions. The choice of interventions is driven by the case conceptualization and should include psychosocial factors such as access to resources. For example, behavioral activation goals such as walking or accessing entertainment resources at a local library may not be feasible for a patient who feels unsafe to walk in their neighborhood. Patients benefit most from behavioral health interventions when they implement them regularly in their daily life. Accordingly, setting goals for how often and when a patient can implement an intervention is important for symptom improvement.

Discussing the goals and limitations of warm handoffs and brief colocated practice with PCPs promotes appropriate referrals and treatment expectations. Having these conversations with new providers to a clinic is especially helpful. PCPs are more likely to think of warm handoffs for patients who present with mental health concerns (primarily suicide risk presentations), and may not recall that some BHPs can help patients with other concerns such as adherence to a diabetes management plan or with interpersonal problems. Department meetings and clinic huddle scenarios are optimal settings to remind providers of the services that BHPs can provide to patients in PC. Patients also benefit from learning about the scope of behavioral health treatment that is offered in their clinic. Pamphlets and TV monitors in clinics can provide helpful information to patients about the behavioral health services that are provided through their PC clinic. Review of consent forms before the start of brief psychotherapy is also a helpful means of communicating the aim and scope of behavioral health treatment in PC.

4.1.1 Interventions

Interventions within IPC are very diverse and vast in number given the number and diversity of presenting problems PC patients have. This chapter will cover some of the common interventions used, but it is not intended to be all-inclusive.

Psychoeducation

Psychoeducation is a component of psychotherapy that is commonly implemented in warm handoffs and brief psychotherapy treatment in PC. It provides BHPs with an opportunity to educate their patients about the common features of mental health diagnoses. Treatment options are also discussed, as well as the course of a disorder. Patients may have their own knowledge base about a diagnosis or have learned about a diagnosis through various platforms or sources such as social media. Through psychoeducation, patients learn accurate information about mental health diagnoses. Patients often describe feeling validated and motivated when they are able to learn how their symptoms are explained by a diagnosis and what they can do to address them.

Psychoeducation also promotes informed decision making

Psychoeducation is most effective when information is presented in a digestible way to patients. Descriptions of mental health diagnoses and terminology used in psychotherapy treatment manuals are typically not going to be comprehended by patients. Thus, BHPs should use terms and examples that the lay community can understand. The words "cognitive" and "behavioral" are commonly used by BHPs and should be defined for patients if they are going to be used in treatment, but preferable words such as thoughts and actions may be substituted. Patients often do not ask for clarification when receiving psychoeducation "blurbs" from BHPs, underscoring the need to be mindful of word choice when delivering psychoeducation interventions.

In PC, BHPs predominantly provide patients with psychoeducation about mental health diagnoses, including generalized anxiety disorder, major depressive disorder, panic disorder, and posttraumatic stress disorder (PTSD). Having a thorough understanding of these disorders and treatment options for them can facilitate the crafting of brief psychoeducation that can be delivered to a patient in less than 1 minute. As with all psychotherapy interventions, it is critical that BHPs assess their patient's comprehension of the information provided through psychoeducation by observing cues such as body language and the patient's ability to reflect back information provided. Patients often do not recall the information discussed with a BHP and thus the use of worksheets with relevant information about mental health diagnoses is helpful.

Care Management

PCPs serve a high number of patients, many of whom have comorbid medical and mental health diagnoses. Delivering services to patients with complex medical and psychiatric presentations can be especially challenging to PCPs who may not have specialized training in mental health assessment and treatment or in methods of building patient relationships such as motivational interviewing. Addressing the needs of patients with complex presentations is also often complicated by psychosocial factors (e.g., lack of access to housing, transportation challenges) and time constraints of PC visits. These patient encounters, often deemed "difficult," are associated with compassion fatigue and feelings of burnout among PCPs.

Care management teams are designed to provide specialized care to patients with complex presentations. These teams include members of different disciplines including PCPs, case managers, nursing staff, pharmacists, and BHPs. Given their training in mental health treatment and interpersonal processes, BHPs can provide valuable support to members of care management teams, as well as behavioral health services to patients with challenging presentations.

BHPs often work on strengthening the relationship between a patient and their care management team, which can become strained due to the complexity of addressing numerous medical and psychiatric concerns. For example, BHPs may provide a private space for both patients and PCPs to talk about their perspectives and emotions with regard to their work together. These interactions can help strengthen the relationship between a patient and PCP and resolve interpersonal conflicts impacting their ability to collaborate.

BHPs can also deliver valuable services to patients with complex medical and psychiatric presentations. Assessments can highlight diagnostic considerations that can inform pharmacological treatment by the PCP and/or suggest referral to additional treatment outside of a PC setting. BHPs can also provide evidence-based behavioral health treatment that can promote the mental health well-being of patients and their ability to adhere to a treatment plan from a PCP.

Working in a case management team can be an invaluable opportunity for BHPs to further strengthen behavioral health integration in their clinic. By design, case management teams are interdisciplinary and function best with an "all hands on deck" approach. They offer BHPs with opportunities to demonstrate the diverse ways in which their skill sets can promote patient outcomes. Team meetings, direct consultations, and didactic presentations are avenues through which BHPs can demonstrate how behavioral health principles and techniques can promote better outcomes and satisfaction for patients and providers.

Relaxation and Meditation Techniques

Relaxation and meditation techniques are commonly introduced to patients in psychotherapy and IPC

Patients are provided with psychoeducation about the benefits of relaxation techniques, how each technique influences the physiological experience of emotions and their body, and the importance of frequent practice to benefit the most from them. Research suggests that relaxation techniques such as deep-breathing techniques are safe and effective for depression, anxiety, stress, and trauma, all of which are common presentations in PC settings (Francesco et al., 2010; Muhammad Khir et al., 2024). Persistent sympathetic activation within the autonomic nervous system is believed to be associated with the experience of distressing emotions (Jerath et al., 2015). Through deep-breathing exercises, parasympathetic activation can dampen the activation of the sympathetic nervous system.

Deep-breathing techniques involve influencing the rhythm of breathing, while meditation techniques are focused on observing naturally occurring processes such as breathing, without manipulation. In deep-breathing exercises, patients are instructed to place one hand on their chest and another on their midsection to better observe how the pacing of deep breathing influences their body. It is important to highlight how overbreathing (involving more chest movement) can further exacerbate feelings of stress and anxiety, while deep breaths (that use the diaphragm muscle) can lessen the experience of such feelings. Patients can practice deep-breathing exercises by sitting down or lying down on the ground on their back. The pace of deep-breathing exercises can be adjusted to the physical abilities of a patient. Most deep-breathing techniques involve breathing in for 4–5 seconds, holding the breath for 2–5 seconds, and breathing out for 4–5 seconds. "Box breathing" is also commonly implemented in PC and consists of breathing in for 4 seconds, holding the breath for 4 seconds, breathing out for 4 seconds, and holding for 4 seconds before breathing in again. Breathing in is predominantly through the nose, while breathing out can be completed through the nose only or a combination of the nose and mouth. Some patients benefit from additional instructions such as telling themselves gently in their own mind to "relax" as they breathe out. Imagery can also be used to help patients get the most out of deep-breathing exercises, including guidance on visualizing one's stress or anxiety exiting the body with every breath that is completed. Deep-breathing exercises can be effective when practiced for 2–5 minutes. The use of an alarm helps patients set a specific time goal for practicing.

An alternative way to teach this breathing exercise would be to teach the patient to do paced breathing. In paced breathing, the patient visualizes in detail that they are holding a flower in one hand and a candle in another. Then, they are instructed to breathe in through their nose and imagine they are smelling the flower and out through their mouth to blow out the candle at 3–4 second intervals for approx. 10 times. This allows the oxygen to carbon dioxide ratio to be recalibrated and calms the body and distracts the mind. Pairing the visualization with the breathing also occupies the mind theregy making it less likely that stressful thoughts occur.

Deep breathing, PMR, and meditation have been shown to be effective in PC settings

Patients often find immediate relief from anxiety and stress through deep-breathing exercises and are thus motivated to practice deep breathing daily, while others may not find the technique as useful. Practicing deep-breathing techniques only during moments of high stress and anxiety will likely not lead to the benefits patients are seeking. Effectiveness of deep-breathing exercises can be augmented by more frequent practice, including during times of relatively low stress and anxiety. An analogy that is useful in describing the benefits of practicing during nonstress times is to explain to patients that we do not teach someone to learn to ride a bike during a hurricane. Rather, they are taught to do so during good weather so their odds of doing so successfully during bad weather improves. BHPs will often provide patients with resources such as online recordings or applications that provide patients with guidance in practicing deep-breathing exercise (see Appendix 2 for resources).

In addition, *progressive muscle relaxation* (PMR) is a valuable tool for relaxation and anxiety and stress management. PMR involves creating tension in muscles and releasing the tension after a short period of time. Muscles that are commonly targeted in PMR include the calves, thighs, biceps, shoulders, and facial and abdominal muscles. Releasing the tension that is created in muscles during a PMR protocol induces relaxation. Patients are instructed to focus on the difference between the feeling of tension in a muscle in comparison with the relaxation that is felt when releasing the tension. Accordingly, PMR involves an attentional component that is similar to meditation practices, yet PMR differs from meditation in that it involves deliberate modification of a physical experience (i.e., tensing muscles), whereas meditation focuses on the attention of a physical process without manipulation of the body. Over time, as more PMR is practiced, patients may develop better awareness of muscle tension in their daily life, which is often an indicator of greater levels of anxiety and stress. PMR protocols vary in length, as some are designed to guide the patient through each individual muscle (e.g., right calf, followed by left calf), versus others that group muscles together (e.g., right and left calves tensed at the same time).

Meditation is another technique that is commonly introduced by BHPs in PC. In meditation, patients practice focusing their attention on internal (e.g., emotions, thoughts, physical sensations) or external (e.g., sounds) stimuli in a manner that is exploratory and without expectation or judgment. During a practice of meditation, attention commonly "wanders" away from the intended target (e.g., observation of breathing without manipulation of the breathing process), and in such circumstances, patients are encouraged to notice when this takes place, and gently redirect their focus to the object of attention. Redirection to the object of attention may need to be completed multiple times during a practice of meditation and becoming distracted should be normalized when guiding a patient through a meditation practice. The nonreactive awareness of internal and external experiences is believed to be the mechanism by which meditation leads to physical relaxation and improved emotional and behavioral management (Lehrer et al., 2007). Specifically, by practicing how to observe and not respond to experiences such as distressing emotions (e.g., anxiety, fear) or thoughts (e.g., self-defeating cognitions) during meditation, patients are able to foster the ability to respond to emotions, cognitions, and physical stimuli in a more mindful, goal-directed manner.

In addition to promoting emotion regulation abilities, mindfulness principles are increasingly used for fostering greater engagement with the present moment. Meditation is believed to improve attentional control abilities that in turn can enhance attention in daily life activities. Better engagement with the present moment may itself reduce experiences of worry and rumination by enhancing the ability to be more "anchored" to the five sensory elements of any given experience. Being able to bring one's attention to the present moment may be especially helpful for individuals with attention deficit disorders or chronic pain, and it can be a helpful component of weight management programs. For example, patients who may be attempting to lose weight and/or foster a better relationship with food tend to benefit from using mindfulness principles when eating – termed "mindful eating." In mindful eating, patients slow down the eating process to more thoroughly experience each food item through the five senses. Savoring and enjoyment of the food item is also promoted, thus enhancing the experience of eating.

Overall, relaxation and meditation techniques are effective for many conditions that patients present to their PCPs and can be introduced in warm handoffs and brief psychotherapy. These techniques are helpful in moments of vulnerability (e.g., panic attacks) and when practiced regularly may improve one's ability to better manage challenging emotions. Mechanisms of relaxation and meditation techniques include changes to the autonomic nervous system and improved functioning of regions of the brain that have been implicated in mental health problems (Hopper et al., 2019; Laborde et al., 2022).

Motivational Interviewing

MI is a person-centered counseling approach that addresses ambivalence for change

Motivational interviewing (MI) is a person-centered counseling approach that addresses ambivalence for change (Miller & Rollnick, 2013). Patients who present to PC settings are commonly ambivalent about a wide range of concerns that are discussed with their PCPs, including coping with a chronic disease (e.g., diabetes) management program that may involve extensive behavioral components (e.g., checking blood sugar levels throughout the day); reducing or eliminating unhealthy behaviors such as smoking cigarettes and unhealthy consumption of alcohol; and starting new health-promoting behaviors like exercise. MI is a person-centered counseling approach that addresses ambivalence for change. MI assumes that individuals are commonly ambivalent about making health behavior changes and helps patients explore the ambivalence in a respectful manner. Talking about ambivalence in MI involves discussing the pros and cons of making a change – this is often surprising to patients, given that most conversations about changing a behavior (e.g., cigarette smoking) focus on the negative elements of the behavior. Fostering motivation in patients is accomplished by discussion of the discrepancy between a patient's current behavior (e.g., smoking cigarettes) and their personal goals for their future. Such discussions foster "change talk" that may resolve a patient's ambivalence and move them toward committing to taking initial steps to address a behavior.

Providers who use MI often cite the importance of using the *spirit* of MI beyond any given MI technique (Miller & Rollnick, 2013). *Rolling with ambivalence*, expressions of empathy, the use of reflective statements, promotion of self-efficacy, and respect for the patient are central elements of this spirit. When using MI, it is important to be mindful of the "righting" reflex which involves the common desire to tell a patient the "right" path they should take to improve their health. MI emphasizes discussion that helps patients describe their own reasons for making a behavioral change. The role of the provider in MI is to review motivational factors, explore potential barriers for change, and collaborate with patients who express readiness to address a particular behavior.

SMART goals are specific, measurable, attainable, realistic, and timely

In MI, once patients have solidified *why* they would want to make a behavioral change, it is important to proceed with developing a plan for *how* a patient will begin to make the change. The use of *specific, measurable, attainable, realistic, timely* (SMART) goals is a helpful guide to creating health behavior change goals for patients (Miller & Rollnick, 2013). Many patients tend to be overly excited or confident in their ability to make a behavioral change, and such expressions should be acknowledged while also encouraging the patient to begin with smaller, more achievable goals. For example, a patient may feel so excited and hopeful about their ability to quit smoking cigarettes upon discussing this behavior with their provider that they may suggest that they will quit their use of cigarettes upon leaving the clinic. Through the use of the SMART goal framework, patients can be encouraged to set more achievable and attainable goals that can set them up for early success with changing a behavior. Providers should document the SMART goal within their encounter note and ensure that they discuss the goal for their next session. Failure to complete SMART goals is to be expected, and exploration of barriers that came up should be completed. Patients may decide that they want to further pursue completion of the SMART goal that they created, or create a more achievable goal. Patient success with SMART goals is often enhanced when all members of patient treatment teams, including the PCP, are supporting patients with SMART goal completion. This kind of team-based approach for behavioral change can provide patients with different perspectives and guidance to complete SMART goals.

As with any other counseling approach, the use of MI does not always lead to commitment to behavior change. It is important for providers to give themselves credit for attempting to use the MI "spirit" and techniques to discuss health behavior changes with their patients regardless of whether it leads to the desired outcome. Implementing MI into one's practice often brings up concerns about the length of time it would take to discuss behavioral change with patients. However, using MI techniques and principles does not necessarily increase the length of sessions and can be highly effective in promoting health behavior change with patients.

Cognitive Behavior Therapy (CBT)

CBT helps patients understand the interplay of emotions, thoughts, behaviors, and physical experiences

Cognitive behavior therapy (CBT) is one of the most widely used psychological interventions and has been shown to be effective for a wide range of mental health problems (Beck et al., 2024). It is a structured approach that aims to help patients understand how their emotions, thoughts, behaviors and physical reactions influence one another over time to drive their experience of a mental health disorder, such as major depression. CBT is based on Aaron Beck's *cognitive theory* which posits that humans develop cognitive structures called *schemas* which inform how they make sense of information around them. The activation of maladaptive schemas is believed to drive the experience of human suffering, including distressing emotions, thoughts, and unhelpful behaviors. The aim of CBT is to develop adaptive cognitions and behaviors that can improve the experience of distressing emotions.

Patients introduced to the CBT framework find it helpful to work with a diagram of the CBT model

Drawing a CBT model on a white board or piece of paper on a clipboard allows BHPs the opportunity to discuss the reciprocal nature of emotions, thoughts, behaviors, and physical reactions with a patient. This also facilitates the discussion of how a patient's experience of a mental health disorder, such as depression, can be conceptualized through the CBT framework. For example, by completing a CBT diagram model, a patient can come to understand how self-defeating thoughts (e.g., "I can never do anything correctly) impacts the experience of emotions (e.g., feeling down), which leads to behavior (e.g., giving up on a work project) that further reinforces self-defeating thoughts and worsens depression.

Behavioral activation is often the first component of CBT introduced to patients. In the CBT model, lack of activity and engagement with the environment, including social relationships, is believed to be a strong contributor to feelings of distress. By working to improve activity levels over time, patients are more likely to develop behavioral habits that promote social reinforcement, positive emotions, and self-fulfillment. First, psychoeducation about behavioral activation is presented to patients, including information on the effects of lack of activity on one's mood. Second, BHPs inquire into possible activities that might interest a patient, especially those that in the past have been reenergizing for them. The importance of engaging in activities each day should be emphasized, as opposed to reserving these activities for vacations or only weekends. Third, reviewing scheduling strategies that enhance the engagement in reenergizing activities is discussed. Patients find it helpful to self-assess their mood before and after completing an activity in order to view firsthand how behavioral activation can improve their mood. It is important for BHPs to highlight that any one given activity is likely not going to substantially improve mood, and that the goal of behavioral activation is to develop the habit of emphasizing consistent engagement in meaningful, reenergizing activities, and that doing so over time can improve mood.

Behavioral activation aims to build a habit of engaging in meaningful activities to improve mood over time

Cognitive restructuring in CBT involves exploration of a patient's maladaptive thoughts and how they are impacting their behavior, experience of emotions, and physical reactions. The cognitive model of depression emphasizes that the characteristic ways in which individuals think will impact their perceptions of the world around them. CBT involves exploration of several cognitions including core beliefs, dysfunctional assumptions, and automatic negative thoughts. *Core beliefs* refer to long-standing, deeply held beliefs about the self, the world, and the future. For example, an individual may believe that they are "faulty" and that the world around them is "unfair." *Conditional assumptions* are conceptualized as rigid rules that individuals adopt that impact their ability to engage in desired behaviors, such as believing that people are never to be trusted. Because of these conditional assumptions individuals engage in *compensatory* strategies, behaviors to compensate for these negative assumptions, which are also often maladaptive. *Automatic negative thoughts* are involuntary thoughts that occur outside the awareness of individuals in certain situations. For example, individuals looking to learn new content or a new skill may experience the automatic thought that they will fail after signing up for a class.

In CBT, cognitive restructuring strategies for maladaptive cognitions include Socratic questioning, completion of thought journal exercises, and directly asking patients for evidence for and against certain thoughts. The overarching goal of these strategies is to develop awareness of unhelpful thought processes and tools for more flexible thinking habits.

CBT often focuses on identifying *cognitive distortions*, defined as unhelpful, irrational thoughts that contribute to maladaptive behavior and distressing emotions (Burns, 1999). Common cognitive distortions include catastrophizing, overgeneralization, all-or-nothing thinking, personalization, mind reading, emotional reasoning, "should" statements, magical thinking, magnification, and minimization. *Catastrophizing* involves the exaggeration of potential consequences of situations (e.g., "If I don't sleep well tonight, I will not function tomorrow at work and I will be fired and then I will be homeless"). *Overgeneralization* occurs when broad conclusions are made from limited events (e.g., I did not do well in my first math test, so I won't do well in any future math tests). *All-or-nothing thinking* involves seeing situations, including oneself, through black and white thinking, without considering the middle or "gray" area (e.g., "I will go every day to the gym for 2 hours, anything less than that is a failure"). *Personalization* refers to holding oneself responsible to events outside of one's control (e.g., "My children are not doing well at their new school. It is entirely my fault."). *Mind reading* occurs when individuals interpret the actions and beliefs of others without evidence (e.g., "My new neighbor did not wave at me this morning, he must not like me"). *Emotional reasoning* involves assuming that emotional experiences are a reflection of the reality of situations (e.g., "I feel uncomfortable in medical school, so I must not belong in medical school"). *"Should" statements* refer to the belief that certain things "should" be a certain way (e.g., "I should have a very clean home every day, if I'm not, I am a failure"). *Magical thinking* involves believing that one's emotions, thoughts, and actions impact unrelated events (e.g., "I thought my coworker would get fired, and because I thought that, he did indeed get fired"). *Magnification* occurs when individuals exaggerate the consequences of events (e.g., "I made a small mistake with a report at work, I bet it will cost me my job"). *Minimization* refers to downplaying the importance of events (e.g., "I was recently promoted at work, but it is not that impressive, everyone gets promoted at some point"). While these are the most common cognitive distortions, others have been identified.

In CBT, cognitive distortions are identified and addressed in several ways. BHP who are trained in CBT may assign thought journals to patients that can highlight cognitive distortions, or may present a worksheet with common cognitive distortions to patients and encourage them to identify the ones that they believe apply to them. Patients may also make statements in therapy sessions that are consistent with cognitive distortions and then these distortions can be addressed when they come up. Interventions for cognitive distortions include directly challenging the distortions as well as coming up with realistic, constructive thoughts for each distortion. For example, in the above example regarding catastrophizing about poor sleep, a patient is encouraged to reflect on whether every time they have had poor nights of sleep they have bad days at work. Additionally, a constructive thought regarding this scenario can be implemented in which a patient reminds themselves that they will likely obtain some sleep and can function reasonably well despite poor sleep. Furthermore, patients are encouraged to explore the situations and contexts in which cognitive distortions occur and to remind themselves of their responses to their cognitive distortions.

In summary, CBT is an evidenced-based psychotherapy for a wide range of mental health disorders. The goal of CBT is to help a patient develop the skills to become their own therapist by equipping them with tools for adaptive behavior and cognitions.

Acceptance and Commitment Therapy (ACT)

ACT is an evidenced-based psychotherapy that aims to promote psychological flexibility

Considered a *third wave* psychotherapy of CBT, *acceptance and commitment therapy* (ACT) emphasizes elements of mindfulness and modifying responses to emotions and thoughts to promote engagement in adaptive behavior (Hayes et al., 1999). ACT builds on CBT's perceived limitations by focusing more on awareness of thoughts and changing one's relationship to those thoughts versus trying to refute them. Clinicians must collaborate with a patient to determine whether CBT or ACT resonates best with them. Third wave therapies like ACT promote acceptance, mindfulness, and values-driven behavior, whereas previous *first wave* and *second wave* therapies focus on behavioral and cognitive restructuring interventions. In ACT, patients are introduced to six processes that promote psychological flexibility, including cognitive diffusion, acceptance, committed action, values, contact with the present moment, and self-as-context. *Cognitive diffusion* refers to the ability to create distance from one's thoughts and emotions so that they do not impact behavior. *Acceptance* is the process by which individuals create space for thoughts and emotions that may be distressing, so that engagement in desired behavior is completed. *Committed action* is the behavior that individuals engage in to move them closer to their desired goals. *Values* refer to the people, actions, and goals that individuals hold important in their lives. *Contact with the present moment* involves noticing whatever processes are happening in any given moment, including thoughts, feelings, and physical sensations that are experienced through the five senses. This process can improve the ability to notice that thoughts, emotions, and physical sensations vary over time and may not consistently be present with the same level of distress. Lastly, *self-as-context*, often termed "the observer self," refers to the ability to take a step back and view the elements of a present moment (i.e., thoughts, feelings, behaviors) with a flexible perspective and ultimately engage in the behavior that is driven by one's values.

ACT can be highly effective in PC settings due to its emphasis on fostering psychological flexibility. Patients in PC tend to present with concerns related to depression, anxiety, trauma exposure, interpersonal problems, and grief; all of which can be addressed through ACT principles and interventions. ACT can be especially helpful for patients in PC who have the goal of completely eliminating their experience of distressing emotions, such as anxiety or chronic pain conditions, by helping them to observe their experience without getting lost in it. Through noticing fluctuations in emotions/thoughts or physical pain sensations, and being able to connect with and make room for all elements of a present moment, ACT can help patients let go of the struggle to eliminate or "control" emotions/thoughts and physical sensations, and instead engage in adaptive behavior. BHPs in PC, due to session limit constraints, often do not have the ability to introduce every ACT intervention to a patient and instead chose the ones that may be most beneficial for patients based on areas of need.

Additionally, CBT and ACT principles may be used in conjunction to promote the well-being of patients. Deciding which intervention to use from each psychotherapy should be driven by the case conceptualization. For example, a patient who presents with grief may benefit from ACT-based interventions to manage the fluctuations of emotions and thoughts related to grief. Over time, cognitive-restructuring strategies from CBT may help the patient challenge maladaptive thoughts related to the passing of their loved one.

PTSD-PC

In addition to depression and anxiety, trauma exposure and PTSD are some of the most common concerns that are addressed by BHPs in PC settings. Warm handoffs may involve addressing recent trauma exposure, and many patients present with anxiety concerns that suggest the presence of generalized anxiety disorder, when in fact their anxiety symptoms are better explained by a diagnosis of PTSD. Accordingly, assessment of trauma exposure and PTSD symptoms can greatly improve the detection of trauma-related disorders in PC. Annual visits with PCPs that involve completion of brief versions of PTSD screening inventories and assessment of trauma exposure when discussing mental health are helpful approaches for the detection of PTSD. For example, the Posttraumatic Stress Disorder Checklist for DSM-5 (PCL-5) will often be administered in PC because it is brief and yet informative about the symptoms a patient may experience after trauma (Weathers et al., 2013).

Trauma exposure and PTSD are some of the most common concerns addressed by BHPs in PC settings

Prolonged exposure (PE) and *cognitive processing therapy* (CPT) for PTSD are two of the most widely used evidence-based psychotherapies for PTSD (Foa et al., 2007; Resick et al., 2024). Until recently, obtaining either PE or CPT for PTSD involved a referral from a PCP or BHP to a specialty mental health facility. Recent research, predominantly in the VHA health care systems, has provided support for brief versions of these psychotherapies in PC settings. For example, a recent study found that a brief version of PE termed *PE for primary care* (PE-PC) was effective in reducing PTSD symptoms among veterans in four to eight 30-minute sessions (Rauch et al., 2023). Interestingly, providers who had prior training in CPT for PTSD and PE were more likely to complete PE-PC cases than those who did not have prior training in PE or CPT, suggesting that prior experience with trauma treatment may be helpful in treating patients with trauma in PC settings and in effectively delivering brief versions of evidence-based psychotherapies for PTSD.

PE and CPT are widely used, evidence-based PTSD treatments

Many patients seek mental health treatment in PC due to the reduced stigma involved with receiving mental health care through PC in comparison with at specialty mental health centers, highlighting the need to provide BHPs in IPC settings with evidence-based brief versions of psychotherapies (Shepardson et al., 2023). Continued research and dissemination of brief versions of psychotherapy for PTSD that can be administered in IPC settings has substantial potential to improve the well-being of patients and lessen the stress of specialty mental health facilities that often have extensive waitlists.

CBT for Insomnia in PC

Chronic insomnia is characterized by early morning awakenings and problems with being able to initiate or maintain sleep. Insomnia is associated with physical and mental health problems including depression, as well as

CBT-I is the first-line treatment for insomnia

economic burden. *Cognitive behavior therapy for insomnia* (CBT-I) is the first-line treatment for insomnia and comprises several interventions designed to improve behavioral and cognitive elements of sleep.

One systematic review that evaluated the effectiveness of CBT-I in PC and community settings could not fully evaluate the effectiveness of CBT-I in PC due to heterogeneity in the setting, program, and assessment of sleep outcomes among studies reviewed (Cheung et al., 2019). However, another systematic review found evidence for effectiveness of CBI-I in PC, with benefits that were maintained several months after treatment concluded (Davidson et al., 2019). Additional research on the effectiveness of CBT-I in PC that includes the use of standardized measures of sleep including daytime functioning assessments is needed. Nonetheless, delivering CBT-I in PC has the potential to greatly impact the health of patients, many of whom will have suffered from insomnia for many years and are looking for solutions that do not involve sleep medications. CBT-I is also a brief intervention (about 4–6 sessions) and thus fits the brief model of care in PC settings.

Insomnia is often comorbid with medical problems, and BHPs can treat this diagnosis in PC settings

Insomnia is believed to be driven by a combination of predisposing (e.g., genetic, hyperactive arousal system), precipitating (e.g., stressful life events), and perpetuating mechanisms (e.g., becoming overly focused on sleep; Spielman et al., 1987). Sleep has also been conceptualized as an automatic process that is disrupted by behaviors such as spending too much time in bed (Espie, 2002). People with insomnia try too hard to sleep and engage in behaviors (e.g., excess worry about sleep, too much time in bed) that cause their experience of insomnia to worsen, leading to significant challenges in daytime functioning such as sleepiness and difficulties with emotion regulation. The goal of CBT-I is to alter maladaptive behaviors that are causing a patient to have sleep problems and begin to develop cognitive strategies that promote psychological flexibility about sleep.

CBT-I treatment comprises several interventions including stimulus control therapy, sleep restriction therapy, sleep hygiene, and cognitive restructuring strategies. *Stimulus control* involves ensuring that patients use their bed for sleep, with sexual activity as the only exception. For people with insomnia, the bed and the bedroom become sources of anxiety and frustration with not being able to fall asleep. These aversive associations are driven by spending too much time in bed while awake and doing other behaviors in the bed and bedroom that do not involve sleep, such as watching television, eating, or worrying. In stimulus control, patients are instructed to go to sleep only when they are feeling sleepy and to get out of bed if they are spending more than 10–15 minutes awake, preferably outside of their bedrooms. Patients are provided with psychoeducation on the difference between feeling sleepy, in comparison with feeling tired, as many tend to go to bed when they are feeling tired but not necessarily sleepy. Tiredness is characterized by feelings of being overly exerted physically (e.g., body soreness), while sleepiness is the state of having difficulties staying awake. Getting out of bed, when not sleeping, while maintaining a commitment to waking up each day at the same time, increases homeostatic sleep drive. Through adherence to stimulus control guidelines, patients come to associate the bed and bedroom with relaxation and sleep. Patients may bring up several concerns related to being able to follow stimulus control guidelines such as space limitations in their homes that restrict the ability to only spend time in their bed or bedroom when sleeping. For such situations, reasonable accommodations can be made that can promote a positive association between sleep and the bed (e.g., instructing college students who live in dorms to go to their dorm desk and read a book if they are having problems falling asleep).

Sleep restriction involves restricting time in bed in order to improve drive for sleep. Patients are instructed to complete a sleep diary to assess various sleep parameters such as how long it takes for them to fall asleep upon going to their bed, awakenings at night and length of them, time spent asleep, and time spent in bed. The restricted window of sleep (time spent in bed) for patients is the average sleep duration based on 1 to 2 weeks of sleep diary data. The wake-up time is kept consistent. For example, a patient whose average sleep duration is 6 hrs and desires to wake up each day at 7:00 a.m. will have a sleep window of 1:00 a.m. to 7:00 a.m. Over time, the patient's sleep window is increased based on subjective feelings of restoration upon awakening. The goal of sleep restriction is to have patients improve their sleep efficiency, which refers to the percentage of time that patients spend in bed asleep. The target sleep efficiency is typically around 80% to 90%, with consistent reporting of good sleep restoration. Importantly, adherence to stimulus control principles during the restricted window of sleep phase is critical to ensure that patients develop a positive relationship with their bed and bedroom. Patients often become concerned about the effects of restricting their sleep window and thus may want to wait to begin sleep restriction therapy on a weekend or during a vacation. There is bound to be discomfort with restricting sleep, and the goal is to endure the short-term discomfort to obtain long-term gains. In general, sleep restriction is an intervention that can help patients improve their sleep on their own and should thus be presented as a set of skills. MI methods may be helpful with getting patients to "buy in" to doing sleep restriction therapy.

Sleep hygiene is a set of strategies and guidelines that promote good quality sleep. The main elements of sleep hygiene involve having a bed and bedroom environment that is quiet, cool, and comfortable, and avoidance of activities that are stimulating before going to bed (e.g., conversations with one's partner about finances). Sleep hygiene guidelines also promote having a relaxing bedtime routine that progressively reduces sources of stimulation (e.g., light from television) and induces physical relaxation (e.g., taking a shower). Patients are instructed to lessen or eliminate the use of substances that may interfere with sleep (such as caffeine) well before the presleep period.

Cognitive restructuring strategies for sleep are also helpful for changing maladaptive thoughts related to sleep. Many individuals with insomnia feel hopeless about their sleep problems and may experience unhelpful thoughts about sleep, especially prior to going to sleep. Helping patients identify, challenge, and restructure such thoughts helps them develop more positive, balanced thoughts about sleep. Additionally, some patients experience performance anxiety related to sleep, such as when attempting to fall asleep. These thoughts are bound to lead to physiological activation that is not conducive to falling asleep and should thus be addressed. Through cognitive therapy for sleep, patients also begin to develop more constructive thoughts about sleep, even on nights in which they may not obtain much sleep. This lessens their experience of catastrophic thinking, such as associating poor sleep on any given night, with poor health or severe bad outcomes during the day.

Overall, CBT-I is an effective intervention for insomnia, a common presentation in PC settings that often exacerbates existing physical and mental health problems. It involves a relatively low number of sessions and is thus a good treatment option in PC. Securing patient commitment to adhering to CBT-I principles and interventions is critical to obtaining the best possible outcomes.

Chronic Pain

Patients frequently endorse difficulties with chronic pain in PC settings. *Chronic pain* refers to persistent bodily pain that lasts for more than 3 months and often involves sensations of aching, burning, shooting pains, squeezing feelings, stinging, or stiffness. Individuals with chronic pain tend to experience difficulties with their mental health, including problems with depression and anxiety. Thus, addressing the mental health challenges of patients with chronic pain can greatly improve their quality of life.

PCPs often consult with BHPs to help patients with chronic pain. BHPs typically complete an initial mental health diagnostic interview that involves a thorough evaluation of chronic pain, including what may have contributed to its onset (e.g., injury or health condition such as arthritis), factors that exacerbate it (e.g., movement, temperature changes, lack of mobility), and interventions that have been previously implemented (e.g., medication, psychotherapy, physical therapy). Patients with chronic pain tend to be skeptical about seeking psychotherapy services for chronic pain because they often fear that they will be told that their experience of chronic pain is "in their head." Accordingly, it is important that BHPs who work with patients with chronic pain conditions are mindful about the psychoeducation they provide patients, including their use of language. Terms such as "complaints" or "catastrophizing" when referring to a patient's experience of chronic pain should be avoided. It is also highly beneficial to provide patients with chronic pain with an opportunity to provide their story of chronic pain, which, due to time constraints, they may not get an opportunity to disclose to other members of their health care team. Providing emotional validation when appropriate can greatly enhance the therapeutic relationship between a BHP and a patient with chronic pain.

Setting specific goals such as improving mobility, mood, sleep, and engagement in meaningful activities (e.g., attending baseball or softball games of loved ones, gardening, attending church services) can improve the effectiveness of psychotherapy for chronic pain. Chronic pain, by definition, is a persistent condition that cannot be fully eliminated, and thus the goal of psychotherapy for chronic pain is to help patients with chronic pain improve their management of the condition. Many patients with chronic pain report their desire to first have their experience of chronic pain improve so that they can engage in more activities in their daily life. Through psychoeducation, BHPs can inform patients with chronic pain that the experience of chronic pain will likely not improve until management of depression, anxiety, and sleep improves and overall mobility increases.

CBT and ACT are used by BHPs to help patients with chronic pain

CBT and ACT are evidence-based psychotherapies for chronic pain (Sturgeon, 2014). BHPs in PC settings typically use elements of CBT and ACT to help patients with chronic pain (Beehler et al., 2024). Interventions that are more frequently used from CBT include paced movement which involves gradually increasing the mobility of a patient with chronic pain, and cognitive-restructuring interventions for thought processes that exacerbate the experience of chronic pain such as *all-or-nothing thinking*. In the context of chronic pain, all-or-nothing thinking can lead to patients engaging in fewer activities due to concerns that the activity (e.g., attending sporting events, going out with friends and family) will not be enjoyed in the same manner as before the onset of chronic pain. CBT-I principles (see the subsection CBT for Insomnia in PC, in Section 4.1.1 Interventions) are also commonly implemented with patients with chronic pain. Improved sleep can greatly enhance the physical experience of chronic pain by providing adequate physical restoration for these patients, as well as enhancing their mood. ACT interventions, due to their emphasis on changing one's relationship with emotional, cognitive, and behavioral experiences that are distressing, are also well received by patients with chronic pain. Discussion of values, and engaging in actions that are consistent with one's values, a central tenant of ACT, are particularly helpful for patients with chronic pain, as they provide them with an opportunity to align their actions with their core values.

Additionally, deep-breathing exercises, meditation, and PMR are interventions that are highly effective for chronic pain management. Educating the patient regarding how muscle tension and lack of oxygen to the muscles can exacerbate pain resulting from nerve damage or other types of physical injuries can increase the likelihood that the patient buys in to the importance of learning breathing and relaxation skills for pain management. As previously discussed in the Relaxation and Meditation Techniques section in Section 4.1.1 Interventions, these interventions are more likely to be effective when used daily, and the effects may not be perceived by patients until they are used for several months. Using these interventions during moments of increased chronic pain in daily life is also highly encouraged. Patients with chronic pain should be frequently reminded that the interventions taught to them will likely not eliminate chronic pain but can improve their ability to manage their experience of chronic pain so that they can engage in activities that they enjoy. The use of MI principles and techniques can also greatly enhance a patient's motivation to adhere to recommended interventions.

Overall, chronic pain is a debilitating condition for many individuals and is a common presentation in PC settings. BHPs can provide patients with chronic pain with multiple interventions that can improve their quality of life. Importantly, helping a patient buy into using these interventions is key to maximizing the benefit they can derive from them.

PCIT is an evidence-based intervention that aims to address disruptive behavior in children ages 2–7

Parent–Child Interaction Therapy (PCIT)

Developed over 40 years ago, *parent–child interaction therapy* (PCIT; Lieneman et al., 2017) has been shown to be effective for several behavioral and externalizing issues. It involves two phases: *child-directed interaction* (CDI) and *parent-directed interaction* (PDI). The goals of CDI are to improve the warmth of the relationship between the parent and the child, increase attention span and prosocial behaviors such as taking turns, and promote more positive interactions. This initial phase of treatment sets the stage for PDI, which directly focuses on addressing the disruptive behaviors of the child. Coaching parents to remain calm as they address the disruptive behaviors of their child is key in PDI.

PC has been deemed as a setting that is highly suitable for parental interventions. A systematic review of parental interventions in PC that assessed child behavioral outcomes found that parental interventions can promote positive outcomes for child behavior (Moon et al., 2020). As discussed earlier, PC settings are often deemed by patients as safer places to seek mental health treatment, and this also applies to seeking parental assistance such that parents may feel more comfortable seeking parental interventions in PC instead of in other specialized mental health settings. Thus, PC may serve as a valuable setting for the provision of parental interventions that can have significant impacts for the mental health of both parents and their young children.

Despite the promise of offering interventions such as PCIT in PC, challenges and questions remain about how to best offer these services. For example, PCIT requires technology such as a live video feed or a one-way mirror and a "bug" in the ear of the parent for the BHP to provide in-the-moment guidance and feedback to the parent as they interact with their child. Thus, PC rooms may need to be adapted to facilitate the delivery of treatments such as PCIT. Additionally, PCIT tends to consist of many more sessions than are typically completed with any given patient in PC. To address this concern, research has investigated the effectiveness of condensed versions of PCIT and has yielded promising results (Graziano et al., 2020). Research that investigates the mechanisms of PCIT has the potential to facilitate condensed versions of PCIT that can more easily be delivered in PC settings.

Problem Solving

A significant proportion of patients in PC settings endorse symptoms of depression, anxiety, and stress. Treatment options for these conditions in PC include medication interventions, for mood and anxiety management, and referral to specialty mental health settings. However, PC patients often prefer to receive assistance for stress and mood difficulties in PC and may also prefer not to be treated via medication interventions. Often, their experience of these symptoms is directly related to a recent stressor in their lives, such as work stress, interpersonal problems, marriage difficulties, problems with parenting, or financial stress. The need to help patients with problem solving and management of depressive and anxiety symptoms prompted the development of *problem-solving therapy for primary care* (PST-PC), a brief psychotherapy that provides patients with skills for solving problems in their lives (Nezu et al., 2013). PST-PC can be delivered individually or in group settings, and it promotes skills that facilitate identifying and solving a current problem. PST-PC involves several modules that promote the therapeutic relationship between the provider and patient, address emotion regulation difficulties that compromise problem solving, and help patients develop problem-solving skills. This form of therapy can be delivered by multiple health care professionals such as PCPs, nursing staff, and BHPs. Research has provided evidence for the effectiveness of PST-PC for anxiety and depressive symptoms (Zhang et al., 2018).

PST-PC involves teaching patients the skills they need to navigate the vicissitudes of life

Additionally, problem solving in PC may be addressed through assessment of stress factors in the lives of patients that can inform targeted intervention for stress management. Stress regulation has been viewed as comprising several components, including stress exposure, stress reactivity, stress recovery, and stress restoration (Williams et al., 2009). *Stress exposure* refers to daily hassles (e.g., interpersonal work stress) and major life events (e.g., birth of child, moving to a different location); *stress reactivity* involves the physiological (e.g., increased heart rate), cognitive (e.g., maladaptive thoughts), and emotional (e.g., anxiety, anger) responses to stress experiences; *stress recovery* is the level of emotional or physiological arousal after the stress exposure ends or the time to reach baseline levels of arousal. *Stress restoration* encompasses processes that promote recovery after stress is terminated, including wound healing and sleep.

Assessment of stress regulation processes can help patients understand their experiences of stress and help practitioners decide which interventions may be more helpful. For example, a patient who presents with anxiety due to constantly missing deadlines, running late for work, and missing important appointments may be conceptualized as encountering stress exposures (e.g., heightened anxiety, interpersonal problems at work, family members who are upset) due to problems with time management. Developing a consistent and sustainable set of organizational skills (e.g., use of planner, alarms on phone) may help with ensuring that problems related to time management lessen stress exposure in daily life. Additionally, stress regulation assessment may highlight the experience of very high reactivity to stress and difficulties getting back to baseline levels, perhaps with reactivity that extends into the presleep period that could negatively impact sleep. In such cases, interventions for physiological stress reduction (e.g., deep-breathing exercises), cognitive restructuring, emotional awareness and acceptance, worry management, and sleep hygiene may address such concerns. Furthermore, stress exposure may be related to interpersonal problems that can be addressed by developing assertive communication skills. In general, assessment of stress regulation can inform which interventions may be better suited for patients in PC based on their experience of stress in their daily lives.

Support and Grief Counseling

Grief is a complex process, and while death of a loved one is often a precursor, individuals may engage in grief in anticipation of a loss, or in relation to losing other valued aspects of life (e.g., mobility, body parts, health functions, social connectedness) or even beloved pets. Below is a discussion related to grief secondary to the death of a loved one, but many of the principles highlighted will apply in other grief scenarios.

The loss of loved ones may involve some of the most stressful times in the lives of people. Grieving processes vary from person to person depending on many factors, such as closeness to the loved one who has passed away, protective factors including social support networks, and mental health history. PCPs often consult with BHPs in situations in which a patient reports struggling with the loss of a loved one. In a warm handoff for grief, BHPs can deliver supportive counseling (e.g., emotional validation) and can introduce techniques (e.g., meditation) for symptom relief. BHPs may also receive referrals for brief outpatient psychotherapy for grief. Some patients experience anticipatory grief when they know that a loved one's prognosis indicates that they likely will not live much longer. Others may experience unexpected deaths that completely change their lives. Regardless of the factors surrounding the death of a loved one, demonstrating compassion, sympathy, and support can be instrumental in helping patients who are undergoing grief. Normalizing the experience of grief can be helpful, as well as providing a safe space to discuss the thoughts and emotions that patients are experiencing related to their grief. Emotions vary for patients with grief and can consist of intense sadness, anger, or happiness. Reassuring patients that experiencing a wide range of emotions, with varying degrees of intensity, is normal when grieving, can be helpful. Most grieving lasts about 1 year, but in some rare cases, individuals may struggle with grief for longer periods of time. Longer periods of debilitating grief may lead to a patient receiving the diagnosis of *prolonged grief disorder* and may require pharmacological interventions and long-term psychotherapy (American Psychiatric Association, 2022).

Patients undergoing grief will benefit from engaging in activities that promote overall activity, such as exercise and spending time with others. Reestablishing routines following the death of a loved one can also help those with grief obtain a sense of normalcy. ACT interventions are especially helpful for patients undergoing grief (see the subsection Acceptance and Commitment Therapy, in Section 4.1.1 Interventions).

Screening, Brief Intervention, and Referral to Treatment

SUDs are common, underscoring the need to develop effective strategies for detection and treatment

PC settings are an optimal setting for the implementation of SBIRT

Screening, brief intervention, and referral to treatment (SBIRT), is a public health approach that was introduced in the 1960s, aiming to identify patients with risky use of substances and provide them with brief interventions and referral to specialty treatment if needed. Patients typically first come into contact with the healthcare system in PC. The growth of validated brief screening tools for alcohol and drug use has facilitated the implementation of screening for *substance use disorders* (SUDs). Many of these screening tools are disseminated to patients through electronic means, reducing the burden of transferring written documentation to the electronic medical chart. Brief interventions in SBIRT involve reviewing of screening results, implementation of MI principles and interventions, and discussion of initial steps to reduce substance use. The SMART goal framework can be used to create an initial substance use reduction goal (see section on motivational interviewing in Section 4.1.1 Interventions). Lastly, a referral to specialty substance use treatment is made when screening results and subsequent discussions with a patient suggest the need for specialized treatment of an SUD.

BHPs in PC may have numerous roles in the implementation of SBIRT. Many spearhead initiatives to imbed screening for SUDs, including alcohol use, into the medical flow of a PC clinic. Additionally, BHPs are often consulted through warm handoffs to facilitate discussions of screening results and provide patients with MI interventions. In some cases, BHPs may also provide psychotherapy to patients that is focused on addressing SUDs.

Numerous studies have provided evidence for the efficacy of SBIRT in PC. Hargraves et al. (2017) provided several suggestions to improve the implementation of SBIRT. They highlighted the importance of including the entire interprofessional team and referral sources in the planning phase of SBIRT, so that everyone can have an opportunity to understand all of the components of SBIRT. The importance of a *practice champion* who can bridge all members of the team was also suggested. The practice champion needs to be someone who is respected and is in a position of leadership, or can receive the support of those who are in positions of leadership within the clinic. SBIRT implementation is also enhanced when members of a PC clinic have a thorough understanding of all of the moving pieces in screening, documentation, and referral processes. Visual flow charts and ongoing training was highly recommended, as well as integration of SBIRT into the electronic health record.

Despite the promising results of SBIRT in PC, ongoing research is needed to increase the effectiveness of SBIRT. Referrals for treatment outcomes are difficult to assess due to limitations imposed by confidentiality, which make it challenging to access treatment outcomes in specialty mental health settings. This barrier highlights the importance of developing and maintaining relationships with referral resources for substance use treatment. Questions have also been raised about the sustainability of SBIRT when grant funding sources end that facilitate the implementation of SBIRT. Nonetheless, SBIRT presents a framework that can help all of those who suffer from SUDs, and it provides BHPs in PC settings with unique opportunities to work alongside an interprofessional team.

4.1.2 Consultations

Patient-Centered Consultations

Patient-centered consultations involve opportunities for BHPs to assist PCPs in delivering care to patients (Cubic, 2019). Such consultations may occur in one-on-one sessions in the clinic and can last from 30 seconds to several minutes or can be initiated via email or messages through the electronic medical chart. The consultation topics vary, from discussions aimed to clarify diagnostics of a patient, to how to best support a patient with difficulties meeting their basic needs.

Regardless of the topic of a patient-centered consultation, it is critical to understand the question or concern of the PCP. This often requires that the BHP ask additional questions to better understand what is known of the patient and what the PCP specifically needs to better understand or needs assistance with to achieve treating a patient effectively. As with warm handoffs, in which information is gathered from the PCP before meeting with a patient, it is critical to read the PCP's body language and the overall situation to ensure that the BHP is not taking up too much time in consulting with the PCP. Succinct feedback and recommendations are best, including offering appropriate resources, if applicable (e.g., referrals for support groups, worksheets that offer psychoeducation, and behavioral health interventions such as deep-breathing interventions).

A common patient care topic that comes up in the context of PC is that of medications for mental health treatment. It is important in such cases for BHPs to be mindful of the limits of their knowledge and training and to be forthcoming about those limitations in their consultations with PCPs. Discussions about opioid and benzodiazepine medications tend to be common in PC, and thus it can be helpful to understand the general policies of the PC clinic with regard to the prescription of these medications. Each PCP is likely going to have a different approach and level of comfort with the prescription of any medication for mental health treatment, and getting a sense of this is highly important to best assist them with treating patients.

BHPs may also be tempted to always have an "answer" for each patient consultation that they have with a PCP. This is not feasible, and it is actually not always going to be the focus of patient consultations. BHPs often provide PCPs with additional considerations about a patient that a PCP may not have thought about or further considered. For example, a patient with consistent low levels of energy and lack of adherence to a medication regimen for diabetes management may be struggling with obstructive sleep apnea which could explain their daytime low energy and problems with managing diabetes. As BHPs are further established within the flow of a PC clinic, they can expect to have more patient-centered consultations. These are great opportunities to build rapport with PCPs and demonstrate the knowledge that BHPs bring to the table in a PC setting.

Provider-Centered Consultations

PCPs typically welcome an opportunity to consult with BHPs when confronted with difficult patients

Provider-centered consultations with BHPs aim to assist the PCP with any concerns they have, such as difficulties in working with patients with a particular presentation (e.g., borderline personality disorder or PTSD) or with some role they may have in their clinic (e.g., training medical students and residents). These consultations can be initiated by the PCP and may also be prompted by someone in a leadership role who believes that a provider needs assistance. Before initiating a provider-centered consultation, it is helpful to discuss the parameters of the consultation, such as limits of confidentiality, especially because the BHP may work with the provider in the future, especially because the BHP may work with the provider in the future. Clarifying these important factors can help a provider feel more comfortable with the consultation. Understanding the *goal* of the consultation is critical in promoting the effectiveness of a provider-centered consultation. For example, a provider may not be seeking "solution" options for a specific set of concerns but instead could be looking for an opportunity to process a particular situation.

Similar to a patient-centered consultation, the BHP in a provider-centered consultation benefits greatly from first understanding what the concerns are of the provider before attempting to offer support. The use of emotional validation and reflections can greatly enhance the interaction. If applicable, a BHP can offer resources to a provider, such as readings that can help the provider with their concern. Offering opportunities for further discussions and support beyond the initial consultation is often well-received by providers.

BHPs may also identify providers in their clinic who may benefit from provider-centered consultations. This is one of the benefits of IPC in that BHPs are working alongside providers and can identify when a provider may benefit from support. These consultations can happen in the trenches of providing patient care and tend to be well received by providers. A demonstration of support, such as recognizing a provider's efforts in treating patients or validation of their emotions, can go a long way in promoting the well-being of providers.

Overall, BHPs often cite that promoting the wellness of their colleagues is one of the most important roles they take on in PC settings and is also one of the most rewarding. Provider-centered consultations present opportunities for BHPs to play an active role in the well-being of their provider colleagues. Being present, curious, and understanding the goal of the interaction are key to ensuring that provider-centered consultations are as helpful as they can be to providers.

Team-Centered Consultations

Due to the team-based nature of PC, BHPs can be consulted to assists teams in their clinic. Examples of *teams* in PC include interdisciplinary teams that consist of multiple providers (e.g., nurses, dietitians, BHPs, pharmacists, physicians) who are providing direct care to patients (e.g., outpatient interdisciplinary clinic for the treatment of diabetes, or an inpatient service); faculty members who train and evaluate family medicine residents and medical students; and specific disciplines such as nurses, physician assistants, nurse practitioners, and clinic support staff who need assistance. In addition, BHPs possess valuable communication skills that can help teams function better.

BHPs are asked to help teams in PC because they are perceived to have the ability to unite team members

Most consultations for teams in PC tend be initiated when something has gone wrong, such as a rift among the members of a team, or in response to some identified issue that the team is looking to address. For example, nursing staff may seek a team consultation from a BHP to gain better understanding of how to effectively help patients who endorse suicidal ideation in the clinic. As with previous consultations discussed, getting a sense of the reason for the team consultation can help BHPs prepare for the consultation.

Team-based consultations can be challenging for multiple reasons. Creating a safe space for honest and open discussion is critical for team consultations but may not be possible if the managers of teams are present for the consultations. Giving everyone in the team an opportunity to voice their perspectives and concerns may be challenging if the team is made up of many individuals, and the consultation is time bound. BHPs may be aware of the concern that prompted the team consultation, yet discussion with the members of the team can reveal additional, perhaps even more concerning, problems than just the original concern. Members of teams may also demonstrate strong emotions during the team consultation or express themselves in ways that are not constructive. There may also be a plethora of perspectives that are expressed, and keeping them together can be very difficult. Lastly, assisting a team that BHPs are a part of can be difficult because members of the team may suspect that the BHP's support is biased.

Despite the challenges of team consultations, BHPs can be effective by attempting to be as prepared as possible before the consultation. Expressing to the members of the team the importance of respecting everyone's perspective is helpful in creating a safe and respectful space for the consultation. If the BHP is a member of the team, it is important to acknowledge it upfront and to be mindful of potential biases that can come up in the consultation. The use of reflective statements aids in members feeling like they are being acknowledged, while giving the BHP an opportunity to better retain the information provided. Reading the room is critical and is often accomplished by noticing the body language, affect, and tone of voice of the members of the team. As the group is expressing feelings, ideas, and concerns, if members of the team appear to be having a constructive dialogue among themselves, the BHP can take a step back and allow the team to move the conversation forward. The BHP can thus function both as a source of information, ideas, and support for the team, and also as a facilitator of a discussion about a particular issue.

Overall, team consultations in PC are bound to come up due to the collaborative, team-based nature of PC settings. These consultations require that BHPs synthesize a great amount of information in a short period of time, with multiple people watching them. Remaining calm and promoting discussion of perspectives and ideas among the members of the team can greatly enhance the effectiveness of team consultations. If needed, scheduling additional opportunities to meet with members of the team may be warranted.

4.2 Development of PC and IPC

4.2.1 Quality Improvement (QI)

QI in primary care aims to enhance the efficiency and effectiveness of patient care

Quality improvement (QI) is a requirement in PC that is intended to promote the efficiency and effectiveness of delivering care to patients. Projects for QI tend to be focused on needs of the community and may be initiated by a needs assessment that identifies an area for improvement. For example, a PC clinic may analyze their own clinic metrics about the patients they serve and notice that a large portion of their female patients have not completed a mammogram in the last year. This observation can catalyze a discussion among members of the clinic to promote the completion of mammograms for the female patients that they serve. Additionally, members of a PC clinic may suggest the need to improve a recurrent process within their clinic, such as the rooming of patients, and such a project would also fall under the umbrella of QI.

QI projects involve different phases. The first phase involves understanding the status quo of a certain area that will be addressed, such as the percentage of patients who complete a colonoscopy, before any initiative to increase the percentage is started. Next, members of the QI project come up with methods and strategies to address the area of focus of the project (e.g., dissemination of messages through the medical chart system to alert eligible patients who have not obtained a colonoscopy). Once the methods and strategies are in place and are implemented, collection of data is completed to evaluate whether there has been a change in the area of interest (e.g., percentage of patients who have completed a colonoscopy after the strategies have been implemented).

A BHP's role in supporting QI initiatives in PC will vary based on the nature of the QI project. If the QI project is one that aims to address behavioral health problems (e.g., improving depression screening and treatment within the clinic), BHPs are often closely involved in the planning, implementation, and evaluation of the project. On the other hand, if the project does not necessarily involve a behavioral health component (e.g., improving colonoscopy completion), BHPs may not play a central role in the QI project. However, they can support the team with various factors (such as consulting on issues related to assessment and measurement, the analyses of data collected, creation of materials for the project such as messages that are disseminated to patients via the medical chart system), and creation of posters, presentations, and manuscripts for journal submission about the QI project.

4.2.2 Program Development

Program development consists of efforts to develop programs in PC to enhance patient care

Similar to the completion of a needs assessment in QI initiatives, *program development* is typically driven by the identification of a need within a population that a PC clinic serves. For example, a PC clinic that serves a high percentage of patients with uncontrolled diabetes and other chronic conditions might develop a program that aims to combine the expertise of various team members (e.g., dietitians, BHPs, pharmacists, physicians, health coaches) to help such patients. The team may decide to create an interdisciplinary clinic to comprehensively help patients with diabetes management or create a program that provides patients with lectures that consist of information and skills for the self-management of chronic illness and promotion of health.

Most programs in PC focus on helping patients improve health behaviors (e.g., exercise, diet, sleep, stress management), and thus BHPs, given their knowledge and experience in promoting healthy behaviors, are often consulted to start the programs. Additionally, BHPs may be consulted to evaluate and enhance an existing PC program. Understanding the history of the program, such as the original needs assessment that drove its development, who the people are who created it, and the manner in which it operates are important to best enhance the program. Such programs are often the "baby" of one or several individuals, so it is important to be mindful of the manner in which feedback and suggestions are made to enhance the program. It is often helpful to begin with describing the elements of the program that are deemed to be good, and to gently describe areas for improvement with suggestions to enhance them.

Program development presents BHPs with opportunities to showcase their talents, yet it is important to note that their development can take a long time and is often met with numerous obstacles. Financial (e.g., reliable continuous source of funding for the program), time (e.g., when to offer patients access to the program during a work week), and logistical (e.g., individuals who can support the logistics of the program) barriers tend to come up when developing a program, and others are identified once it is started. Supporting colleagues who are working to start and enhance a program can be a big role for BHPs in program development.

Overall, program development is an exciting opportunity for BHPs to use their skill sets to create programs that can positively impact the health of patients in their community. PC clinics often showcase their programs on their websites or publish articles describing their programs. These resources can help BHPs better understand how other PC clinics have developed their programs and can thus serve as a launching base for their own efforts to start programs in their clinic.

4.2.3 Pitching IPC to Leadership

Anyone working in a PC setting has to be aware of funding realities and the need for strategic allocation or resources

PC leaders work diligently to balance high-quality care, provider satisfaction, and the finances of their setting: In short, "No money, no mission." Therefore, a PC practice must thoughtfully transition to IPC. Advocates for IPC are best served by preparing a business plan prior to pitching the concept of a practice transitioning to a more integrated model. Ideally, a needs assessment would also have been performed to provide an even more compelling argument for how integrating behavioral and medical services would be beneficial to the patient population, providers who serve them, and the clinic or institution.

Because there is almost universal agreement that integrating behavioral health services into PC settings is beneficial in numerous ways, data from numerous studies (Archer et al., 2012; Nederveld et al., 2023; Reiss-Brennan et al., 2016; Schmidt et al., 2018) can be used to start the conversation and get leaders interested in exploring possibilities. The logistics of creating and sustaining IPC, however, can be challenging and require support from upper management and leadership. The most typical barrier to integration is determining payment models that will cover integrated types of services.

Financial managers for institutions and practices are often concerned that an integrated model is not financially viable in the long run. Furthermore, within the United States, the fact that states have varying types of health care systems and payment structures and plans makes it even more complicated. Additionally, each state's payment models vary across insurance providers and contracts, making integrated care even more complicated.

Quality IPC has critical components, such as collaboration and communication between team members; however, for the most part, current insurers will not pay for any of the time required to do these activities. Additionally, many payers will not reimburse two different health professionals providing a service to the same patient on the same day. Consequently, IPC varies from state to state, depending on many factors related to how that state reimburses mental and physical health services and other rules and regulations related to it. It also appears inevitable that clinics located in rural settings are less likely to have IPC, because it is more challenging for them to recruit BHPs.

In our health care system paying for IPC continues to be a challenge

Subsequently, there are no *one size fits all* recommendations that can be made. It is recommended that BHPs educate themselves about business matters related to the practice into which they would be integrating. This would include gaining an understanding of their state's reimbursement challenges and opportunities. The clinic should also see these issues – that is, payment models – as part of the needs assessment process.

4.2.4 Integrating IPC Principles Into Educational Programs

Interprofessional Opportunities

The reality is that most health care professionals, whether in IPC or not, will work in settings with many other types of disciplines other than their own. However, many health care professionals train in silos, which make it much harder for them to be able to work effectively within team-based care models, such as IPC. Therefore, the value of interprofessional education has been increasingly recognized. As discussed earlier (see Section 1.3 Competencies Needed), this recognition has led to the creation of core competencies for interprofessional collaborative practice that were updated in 2023 (IPEC, 2023). This IPEC workgroup acknowledged that if didactic and experiential interprofessional training opportunities occur, health care professionals value the role of others from different health care professions with whom they will work throughout their careers. Unfortunately, despite the increased demand for BHPs in PC, training programs in mental health fields typically do not offer coursework or practicums in IPC settings. Surveys have shown that behavioral health training programs that do offer training in IPC often do not offer it as a major course of study (Cubic & Beacham, 2014; Cubic et al., 2011). Additionally, while medical students and residents often train with nurses and other health care providers, they may have limited interprofessional training with BHPs. In fact, most medical students only receive training regarding mental health as part of their third-year clerkship with psychiatry, which often occurs in inpatient psychiatric settings. Directors of family medicine residency programs have also recognized the need for residents to have more interprofessional training opportunities (Green et al., 2022).

Training programs need to develop a strategic plan for education and training to prepare the upcoming workforce

BHP training programs have to address predictable attitudinal, financial, clinical and operational barriers. This training needs to focus on helping trainees cultivate the skills and competencies that promote collaboration among the health disciplines. Attitudes formed early in educational training can have long-lasting impacts throughout a professional career; therefore, academic departments should encourage collaboration through didactic education and interprofessional training (Cubic et al., 2012; Serrano et al., 2017).

For example, family medicine residencies have traditionally been required to have faculty members dedicated to the integration of behavioral health. Most frequently, this has been a BHP, but there has been no uniformity in how this is accomplished. Some BHPs only provide didactics on behavioral health topics, while others only oversee observational experiences for family medicine residents (e.g., a resident observing a psychiatrist, psychologist, social worker, etc.). This has seldom meant that family medicine residents work side-by-side clinically with BHPs on a regular basis. However, an opportunity is on the horizon. New Accreditation Council for Graduate Medical Education (ACGME) guidelines for family medicine residencies disseminated in 2023 have promoted IPC as an expected portion of the resident's training experience (Accreditation Council for Graduate Medical Education, 2023).

An example on the BHP side, where the importance of interprofessional training has been recognized, would be psychology. The American Psychological Association has noted that improvements can occur to facilitate an exchange in training between fields such as medicine and psychology. To do so, psychology departments must modify how they provide educational and hands-on clinical experiences to trainees (Bluestein & Cubic, 2009; Cubic & Beacham, 2014). As PC is often the first point of contact for addressing mental health problems, psychologists training within a PC setting may be required to provide treatment to a demographically diverse population, with a wide range of psychological concerns with varying severity. Moreover, given the fast-paced nature of PC, psychologists working in this setting may be responsible for a sizeable client load and will need to learn the skills associated with brief assessments and treatments. Because these differences between IPC and traditional psychological practice require unique skills, training programs must adequately prepare psychology trainees to practice in IPC settings (Bluestein & Cubic, 2009).

Didactic Resources

While interprofessional training opportunities are necessary to prepare trainees to work in IPC settings, didactic coursework is also required to give them the knowledge base to be successful. The fields of psychology and social work have each created curricula that can be utilized by faculty in graduate programs to introduce IPC to trainees and teach them the fundamental principles associated with working in PC settings. Below we discuss an example of one of these curricula.

The American Psychological Association's Society for Health Psychology's Committee on Integrated Primary Care developed a training curriculum (Ward-Zimmerman et al., 2017), which was supported by research on training (Stillman et al., 2018) and can be used by graduate programs to train on IPC. The curriculum titled, *Integrated Primary Care Psychology: An Introductory Curriculum*, was designed primarily to provide trainees with foundational skills for IPC. The comprehensive *plug and play* design of the curriculum was created by nine psychologists with extensive experience and backgrounds in IPC. The curriculum is comprised of four foundational modules (available in a 90-minute or 120-minute version) as well as 18 topic modules (90-minute version). The four foundational modules focus on the basics of understanding the competencies required for working effectively in IPC. These are listed in Table 1. The modules use illustrations, videos, interactive exercises, and the latest empirical support to cover topics including the role of psychology in PC, PC patient needs, common health concerns in a PC setting, and the application of clinical skills in PC. Table 2 lists and describes the 18 specialized topic modules that focus on common mental health issues seen in PC, including depression, anxiety, trauma, substance abuse, and chronic pain.

Table 1
Four Foundational Modules From the Integrated Primary Care Psychology: An Introductory Curriculum

Foundational modules		Topics covered
Module 1	Introduction to integrated primary care	Defines the field, identifies key factors leading to integration, and discerns the role of the traditional mental health provider to the role of the psychologist in primary care
Module 2	Across the continuum: Psychology's role in IPC	Discusses the range of patient needs presented in primary care
Module 3	Primary care patients: Who are they and how can psychologists be helpful?	Describes common patient behavioral health concerns in primary care
Module 4	IPC interventions	Identifies the clinical skills associated with providing interventions suited for primary care

Note. IPC = integrated primary care. Adapted from Ward-Zimmerman, et al., 2017.

Table 2
Specialty Topic Modules From the Integrated Primary Care Psychology: An Introductory Curriculum

Specialty modules		**Topics covered**
Module 1	Anxiety disorders in IPC	Presents the prevalence rates of patient anxiety in PC and its impact; screening; processes; intervention approaches; strategies for family engagement and how to consult with the PCP
Module 2	Attention-deficit/ hyperactive disorder (ADHD)	Discusses symptoms of ADHD present in PC across the life span and how psychologists can improve identification and treatment of ADHD
Module 3	Chronic disease	Describes successful chronic disease self-management across the lifespan; psychological factors associated with chronic medical diseases; and psychological interventions that promote chronic disease self-management skills
Module 4	Chronic pain	Illustrates how pain presents in PC; the biomedical and biopsychosocial models of pain; and chronic pain assessment, screening, and interventions addressed in PC
Module 5	Depression	Presents depression prevalence rates in PC and its impact, the relationships between depression and health and health care utilization; key studies demonstrating the effect of the collaborative treatment approach to depression; and best practices in depression screening and intervention
Module 6	Health promotion and disease prevention	Covers the BHPs role in health promotion; screening instruments used to detect risk for behavioral health disorders; and interdisciplinary disease management interventions
Module 7	Motivational enhancement strategies	Describes the essential elements of motivational interviewing (MI) and brief action planning (BAP) and how to apply MI and BAP concepts to patient care
Module 8	Older adults	Discusses typical behavioral health issues in older adults; evidence-based mental health treatment for older adults; and tools used for brief cognitive assessment
Module 9	Psychologists as scientists in IPC	Reviews research skills needed in PC; characteristics of dissemination and implementation (D&I) science; and how D&I science helps evaluate outcomes in health care
Module 10	Substance misuse	Presents the prevalence and presentation of substance use and misuse in PC; strategies for preventing and managing substance misuse; and information about SBIRT
Module 11	Training trajectory	Underscores the competencies needed to work in IPC; key differences between traditional and integrated training settings; and the types of questions trainees need to ask to identify IPC training opportunities
Module 12	Cognitive difficulties	Presents the prevalence rates of cognitive issues in PC and their impact; screening and intervention approaches; strategies for family engagement; and how to consult with the PCP

Table 2 Continued

Specialty modules		Topics covered
Module 13	Pediatric chronic pain	Illustrates how chronic pain presents in pediatric settings and chronic pain assessment; screening; and interventions which have been modified for children and adolescents
Module 14	Pediatric primary care	Underscores the similarities and the differences between IPC in pediatric settings versus those in adult and geriatric settings
Module 15	Posttraumatic stress disorder (PTSD)	Presents the prevalence rates of patients presenting with PTSD and trauma in PC and its impact; screening and intervention approaches; strategies for family engagement and how to consult with the PCP
Module 16	Introduction to SBIRT	Provides details about SBIRT model of care and how to best implement it in PC settings as well as data to support its effectiveness
Module 17	Symptoms that defy diagnosis	Reviews patient presentations that are difficult to diagnose and treat and ways to maintain compassion for patients that defy the development of straightforward treatment plans
Module 18	Trauma-informed IPC	Illustrates the importance of interdisciplinary collaboration in providing trauma-informed care across PC settings

Note. BHP = behavioral health provider; IPC = integrated primary care; PC = primary care; PCP = primary care provider; SBIRT = screening, brief intervention, and referral to treatment. Adapted from Ward-Zimmerman et al, 2017.

4.3 Efficacy and Prognosis of IPC

IPC improves access, enhances care, boosts job satisfaction, and reduces costs

IPC is associated with increased access to care, improved patient outcomes, higher job satisfaction for those who work in an IPC setting, and decreased health-related costs (Archer et al., 2012; Fraser et al., 2018; Nederveld et al., 2023; Reiss-Brennan et al., 2016; Schmidt et al., 2018). Much of the research on IPC has consisted of studies that evaluate the effectiveness of the PCBH model (see Section 2.2.1 Primary Care Behavioral Health). One systematic review found that the PCBH model is associated with improved patient outcomes (e.g., depressive, anxiety symptoms) and greater access and utilization of behavioral health services, both within PC and specialty mental health care (Possemato et al., 2018). This review highlighted methodological issues that limit the ability to fully evaluate the effectiveness of the PCBH model. Nonetheless, the evidence for the effectiveness of IPC is strong, in particular for depression and anxiety, two of the most common diagnoses that are addressed in a PC setting.

As more health care systems have adopted the IPC model, the need to evaluate its effectiveness has increased. IPC, as a model of care, is appealing to patients and providers, yet research that aims to examine the mechanisms of its effectiveness is lacking. This may ultimately impact whether health care systems implement IPC in the future and whether systems that currently have an IPC model continue to allocate resources to maintain its existence.

Funderburk and colleagues (2024) highlighted the importance of conducting future research that evaluates the effectiveness of IPC models, specifically PCBH components that lead to patient behavioral changes. They argue that past research supports the effectiveness of behavioral interventions helping specific populations within an integrated model of care, and that there is a need to better understand the effectiveness (e.g., mechanisms of change for patients) of the broad model of PCBH. As patients progress through different stages of the PCBH model (initiation of care, assessment and action planning, behavioral health service provision), mechanisms driving patient behavioral change are proposed. For example, in the initiation of care pathway stage, a patient who is introduced to a BHP by their PCP is able to see firsthand that PCBH care that is provided by a BHP is standard within their PC clinic. The introduction by the PCP may also improve the credibility of the PCBH model and the BHP, as well as the patient's receptivity to PCBH services. Understanding which of these mechanisms leads to patient change (e.g., willingness to attend an initial behavioral health appointment) can support efforts to enhance the effectiveness of IPC.

4.4 Variations of IPC Method and Combination With Other Approaches

4.4.1 Facilitating Specialty Care

Helping patients get connected with specialty care is a hallmark of IPC

There are numerous ways in which patients who obtain health care services in PC may be transitioned to specialty care in the community. Warm handoff encounters may lead to BHPs deciding that the best course of treatment for a patient is to begin specialty care as soon as possible. Initial diagnostic assessments with patients can also reveal that the patient's mental health concerns are outside of the scope of what can be effectively addressed in a PC setting and thus suggest the need to refer to specialty care. BHPs greatly benefit from having a general sense of the kinds of specialty mental health services that are available within their own health care system and community to facilitate such referrals. Patients need to be provided with thorough rationales for why they would benefit best from receiving specialty mental health care instead of obtaining behavioral health treatment in a PC setting. It is common for BHPs in PC to see patients for several sessions before a patient is able to transition to specialty care.

Referring to specialty care can be impacted by numerous factors. Lack of specialty clinics within the community, long waitlists, medical insurance barriers, and transportation difficulties are some of the many roadblocks to transitioning patients to specialty care. Additionally, a patient may not follow up with attending services offered by a specialty mental health facility, due to the mental health stigma related to receiving specialty mental health care. Openly talking to patients about these concerns and potential barriers is crucial to bridging them to the care that they need. BHPs typically keep a working list of referrals for specialty care in the community and categorize them based on the medical insurances they accept. The latter component can at times change without notice on specialty care websites, and thus patients should be encouraged to consult with specialty care facilities to ensure that they accept their medical insurance.

In addition, patients may follow through with receiving specialty care if they can have an appointment set up with the specialty care facility. For example, in a warm handoff scenario, it can be helpful to have a patient reach out to a specialty care facility (e.g., long-term psychotherapy in private practice) and set up an appointment while the BHP remains in the room with them. This can help patients feel like there is a clear path from seeing their providers in PC and transitioning to a specialty mental health care service.

4.4.2 Utilization of Technology and AI in IPC

AI has significant potential to improve health care processes and patient outcomes

The tremendous potential for *artificial intelligence* (AI) to enhance health care system processes and patient outcomes has become significant and salient in recent years. AI refers to technology that has the ability to perform processes, such as reasoning, in ways that humans can. In IPC, the potential of AI is intriguing given the demands of operating as a BHP in PC. Assistance with completing documentation (e.g., warm handoff notes), diagnostic decision making following a behavioral health intake session, deciding what intervention (e.g., CBT vs. ACT) may work best for a patient given their presenting concerns, and ecological momentary interventions outside of traditional psychotherapy sessions are some of the ways that AI can enhance the effectiveness and efficiency of BHPs in PC (Gual-Montolio et al., 2022).

The power of AI lies in its ability to synthesize vast amounts of data, beyond the capabilities of the human brain. This output of data can inform processes that impact the practice of BHPs in PC. For example, AI technology may be able to assist BHPs in PC with being able to synthesize a vast amount of data from a medical chart (e.g., age, race, medical diagnoses, medications, past surgical interventions, blood pressure history) that can inform assessment and interventions in a warm handoff scenario. Additionally, data gathered throughout the course of psychotherapy treatment that is processed through AI technology can inform treatment strategies by BHPs.

Despite the promise of AI, many questions remain about how to safely and effectively use AI to promote the wellness of the public. Perhaps the biggest concern is that AI used to provide psychotherapy services may become so advanced and sophisticated that it may end up replacing BHPs. However, despite the promise of AI assisting psychotherapy processes (e.g., diagnostic decision making, ecological momentary assistance throughout psychotherapy treatment), AI is likely not going to be able to provide empathy to patients, which is a central element of psychotherapy (Rubin et al.,

2024). Empathy and the human connection are critical mechanisms that drive the effectiveness of psychotherapy and are unlikely to be replaced by AI technology.

Overall, AI in IPC has great potential, yet caution should be exercised when using this form of technology. Output from AI (e.g., drafts of diagnostic evaluation reports, diagnostic impressions, treatment recommendations) can serve as an initial starting point for tasks that are routinely completed by BHPs, but should not be automatically used without thorough evaluation of the output. AI, like any form of technology used by health care professionals, should be used as a tool, with the ultimate clinical decisions resting in the hands of the human professional. As AI technology is increasingly incorporated in PC, BHPs may benefit from being present in discussions and implementation efforts of AI to ensure that the adoption of AI does indeed meaningfully facilitate the practice of BHPs in PC.

4.5 Problems in Carrying Out Treatments

4.5.1 Patient Acceptance

Patient buy-in is critical to the successful implementation of IPC. Any given provider, regardless of their training background, will not be effective if their patients are not invested in their suggested treatment plan. It can be easy to see patients as a collection of diagnoses, demographics, and presenting "complaints," yet it is pivotal to see patients as individuals with lives, aspirations, dreams, and concerns that can indeed be very distressing. The high volume of patients that are seen in PC clinics, and other factors such as burnout, compassion fatigue, and at times limited access to resources, contribute to not seeing patients as the complex individuals they are. Reminding oneself to attempt to explore the humanity of the people that come into one's clinic can greatly enhance patient acceptance of behavioral health.

The social psychological literature has found that humans have an innate ability to detect when someone is genuine and trustworthy. This "gut instinct" that humans are equipped with tends to be right most of the time. As a result, being able to be *present* with the patients is pivotal to obtaining their buy-in. Much of how people discern whether someone is truly invested in their care lies in their ability to read body language cues. Behaviors, such as clicking one's pen while seeing a patient, spending too much time on the medical chart, lack of eye contact with a patient, and having a "one foot in, one foot out" approach to care will likely lead to a patient feeling like they are not receiving the care they are looking for. Being present, empathetic, and honest with patients can be critical to obtaining patient buy-in. Interventions such as MI and implementation of positive reinforcement can also build commitment to adherence to a suggested intervention. Overall, patients often do not always remember what providers tell them, but they do recall the overall feeling of the interaction.

BHPs tend to obtain training that focuses on establishing rapport with patients, yet the nature of operating in a PC setting – mainly the high volume of patients that are seen – can compromise a BHP's ability to be present and empathetic with their patients. Meditation, five sensory grounding techniques, and interventions that target physiological symptoms of anxiety (e.g., deep-breathing exercises, PMR) can help BHPs be present with their patients. Using such interventions throughout the day, such as during the lunch hour or short periods of time, before transitioning from one patient to the next, can be beneficial. BHPs in PC often play numerous roles in their clinic, including mentoring and supervising students, teaching, and participation in committees. Having these roles and responsibilities within a PC clinic can give BHPs the opportunity to use their diverse skill sets and may also serve as a reset from the wear and tear of delivering patient care.

BHPs can often benefit from periods of deep breathing, PMR, or meditation while they guide patients in these activities

In addition, the process of a warm handoff can greatly enhance patient's willingness to obtain behavioral health services. In a warm handoff, the PCP introduces the BHP to the patient and vouches for the services that the BHP can provide to the patient. This process puts a "face" to the BHP, thereby increasing the likelihood that the patient will adhere to behavioral health treatment recommendations and follow-up visits if applicable.

4.5.2 Provider Buy-In

PCPs run busy practices and are often juggling numerous professional responsibilities. Bluestein and Cubic (2009) described introducing behavioral health trainees who are new to the IPC model, to the "When in Rome, do as the Romans do" philosophy that highlights the importance of BHPs needing to adapt their style, practice, and documentation to that of the PC setting. The integration of BHPs into the flow, pace, and culture of PC takes time, yet is critical to earning the trust of PCPs. For example, PCPs may not recognize the challenges posed by dual relationships for BHPs or may see BHPs as only necessary when significant mental health concerns arise for their patients, such as suicide risk, as opposed to being aware that the BHP could assist with treatment adherence, pain management, sleep improvement, or a variety of other issues. The more a BHP operates effectively as a PCP, the more likely they will be thought of as a helpful resource for patients.

Working in PC as a BHP requires assimilation into the flow and culture of PC

Providing education to physicians about the scope of practice of a BHP in PC is key to ensuring that over time physicians best utilize behavioral health resources within their clinic. Physicians often do not know the ethical standards that BHPs have to adhere to or even the kinds of services and interventions that BHPs can provide to patients. Providing physicians with small blurbs of education on these matters can facilitate collaboration in the long-term. Moreover, BHPs can greatly benefit from understanding the mindset and workday flow of their physician colleagues. Gaining an understanding of the numerous factors that PCPs take into consideration when treating patients (e.g., diagnoses, billing, insurance coverage) can help BHPs better deliver information, whether orally or through written documentation, that can be efficiently incorporated into what providers are considering for any given patient.

At a more basic level, providers will come to trust BHPs when they receive positive feedback from their patients about the services they are receiving from BHPs. Some physicians may be skeptical about the role that behavioral health services can play in supporting their patients, and these perceptions are challenged when patients themselves report the benefits they are obtaining from their BHPs. Most BHPs will at some point encounter a provider who is highly resistant to consulting them to help their patients, and in such cases, there may not be much that can be done to change the mentality of the provider. However, if the BHP gets an opportunity to intervene, even once, with a patient that a PCP is having difficulty managing successfully and is able to make a difference, the PCP could be swayed to value IPC more.

4.5.3 Pacing in Primary Care

PC clinics are very busy settings that aim to provide the highest quality care to the greatest number of patients possible. In other words, PC clinics operate on a population-based model with a goal of providing a broad array of services to a large number of patients as opposed to specialty clinics which can provide more in-depth services but only to a limited number of patients. BHPs have to operate at the same pace as their provider colleagues to be the most effective. Most BHPs are trained in their home programs in significantly different settings than PC. Thus, the learning curve to translate the fundamental knowledge and skills that BHPs learn to PC settings can be steep.

The key to this transition is learning to be flexible. In the world of PC, BHPs' schedules are fluid and can change quickly. Very seldom do they have days that unfold exactly how they planned them. In any given hour, a BHP may go from completing a warm handoff to supporting a trainee, and finishing with a discussion with leadership about an operations concern, all while needing to complete documentation for the warm handoff. Over time, the frantic nature of PC clinics tends to slow down and becomes the new normal.

The best way to learn about the pacing of PC is to observe the operations of a PC clinic first hand. A lot occurs between a patient checking in at the front desk and ultimately checking out upon completion of their visit. Special attention should be paid to the nature of communication between all members of a PC clinic, which tends to be goal-directed and in bullet-point form. Understanding what each member of a PC team has to do on the medical chart to document and close an encounter is especially valuable. Shadowing PC visits and when possible, provider procedures, can highlight the nature of concerns that are addressed by providers and the time they allocate to each patient.

It is important to note that working in PC is not a good fit for everyone. Elements of one's personality, comfort with unpredictability, and career aspirations play a role in the setting that BHPs choose to work in. BHPs, who work in PC settings, frequently cite the fact that they enjoy having days that are eclectic and fast-paced, and the opportunity to collaborate with members of a PC team. Shadowing and training in PC can provide BHPs with a glimpse into how their workdays would be should they decide to work in PC. In addition, not all PC clinics operate in the same manner. Any given clinic has its own culture and overarching goals. For example, some PC clinics are independent businesses, while others may have a residency program that plays a major role in how the clinic operates. Some PC clinics have robust programs of research, while others may not emphasize research. Thus, BHPs should seek employment at PC clinics that align with their own respective goals and aspirations.

4.5.4 Time

Due to the fast-paced nature of PC, working as a BHP in a PC setting requires efficient use of time

The overarching goal of IPC is to provide effective behavioral health services to patients in PC care in a limited time frame. To do so, in the context of providing behavioral health services such as assessments and interventions, BHPs need to quickly collect and synthesize information, make decisions that are accurate and evidence-based, and deliver feedback and interventions that are effective in a short time frame. BHPs in PC benefit from developing an "internal clock" that helps them check in with themselves about how much time they have spent on any given component of a patient interaction. For example, in the context of a warm handoff, establishing rapport with a patient may involve asking a patient what they did during the past weekend or a recent holiday. Such discussions cannot be so extensive that they compromise the BHP's time to address the referring provider's consultation concerns. Thus, being able to gently redirect patients is critical to ensuring that warm handoffs and brief psychotherapy interventions are effective. Reflective statements that summarize what a patient has said and end with a redirection (e.g., new question, observation, psychoeducation) are especially helpful.

Interventions must also be adapted in order to be delivered in a more condensed manner with the essential elements of the intervention. Many BHPs in PC contexts save a lot of time when working with patients by having a collection of *worksheets* that they provide patients, which contain psychoeducation about mental health diagnoses and interventions, guidance on practicing techniques, and resources to access helpful mental health tools online. The use of these worksheets can greatly help BHPs use their time more efficiently in patient encounters. An overview of resources with worksheets and handouts is provided in Appendix 2. An overview of some commonly recommended apps for behavioral health is provided in Appendix 3. In addition, documentation in PC settings tends to be extensive and time consuming. Developing tools and shortcuts for documentation completion within the medical chart system can greatly enhance efficiency and save time. Such tools may include note templates for different kinds of patient encounters (e.g., intake sessions, warm handoffs) and organization systems to keep track of clinic or department activities (e.g., committee meeting times, teaching obligations).

No-show patients free up BHP time for notes and other necessary tasks

The IPC model often leads to time gaps during the day of a BHP. These time gaps may occur due to the delivery of brief psychotherapy, no-shows by patients, or while teaching, precepting practicum student and interns, or collaborating with PC team members in an interdisciplinary clinic. These are critical times gaps for BHPs to complete patient encounter documentation and other relevant clinic activities (e.g., checking patient inbox, responding to and sending emails, reviewing materials for teaching). Even starting a patient encounter note during a brief 2- to 3-minute period before moving on to the next task can help BHPs wrap up their workday in a timely manner. In general, it is highly beneficial to use time efficiently when working as a BHP in PC.

Many philosophies, quotes, and sayings can be applied to working in PC. Legendary UCLA basketball coach John Wooden once said, "Be quick, but don't hurry." This quote applies to the world of IPC. BHPs must indeed be quick in their decision making, synthesis of information, and delivery of services, all while not rushing any given aspect of what they do. Rushing, especially when working with patients, compromises the overarching goal of delivering high-quality care to patients.

4.5.5 Challenges in Coordination

Challenges in the coordination of delivering behavioral health services to patients are common in PC. These challenges in coordination are likely impacted by each PC clinics' location, structure, resources, and populations they serve. In general, staff turnover that has a negative impact on the coordination of patient care, errors in appointment scheduling, and room availability are some of the common challenges that BHPs face when attempting to deliver care to patients. Many of these coordination challenges can be mitigated by the implementation of workflows that facilitate behavioral health referrals within the medical chart, communication systems to alert BHPs of a warm handoff request, and designation of an office space that is reserved for behavioral health services. As with the establishment of a SBIRT model in PC, visual diagrams that help every member of a PC team understand the process by which patients are scheduled and treated by BHPs can help everyone be on the same page.

Importantly, BHPs in PC often need to collaborate with members of a PC team, such as nursing staff, to ultimately be able to see patients in need of behavioral health services. These collaborations are aided by getting to know nursing staff and other coordinators who have an understanding of available resources (e.g., rooms). Communication with these PC team members should be succinct and respectful. Thanking them for their help after completing a patient encounter can greatly aid in establishing rapport and enhancing their willingness to help in future situations. When conflicts arise in the coordination of care, approaching the members of the PC team who can help with a sense of curiosity and a desire to understand what may be driving the conflict, can promote better outcomes.

4.5.6 Barriers Regarding Billing of IPC Interventions

The evidence base for IPC is very intriguing, yet the billing of IPC interventions is challenging

The increase in mental health problems has led to the increased incorporation of IPC by numerous health care systems and independent PC clinics. However, billing for IPC continues to be problematic for those looking to bring behavioral health integration into their practice. A recent study of 44 practices found that behavioral health integration was funded through numerous combinations of payment strategies, and that these varied based on hospital affiliation status (Ma et al., 2022). This study indicated that hospital-affiliated practices were more likely to fund integrated behavioral health services via pay-for-performance and fee-for-service incentives, whereas non-hospital-affiliated practices tended to use support from grants or other general medical education funds. It was suggested that practices that use grants and general medication education funds to support behavioral health integration may struggle with sustainably funding for IPC services, given the fluctuating and challenging nature of obtaining such funding. Accordingly, finding a pathway for sustainably funding IPC is critical to incorporating and maintaining behavioral health integration in PC.

Behavioral health integration services that are provided in a PC setting vary, and they impact how a PC practice may be able to fund IPC. Elements of IPC that resemble those of an outpatient independent psychotherapy practice (e.g., intake diagnostic sessions, follow-up psychotherapy sessions, assessments for disorders such as ADHD) are often easier to charge for than components of IPC such as warm handoffs.

4.6 Multicultural Issues

4.6.1 Cultural Awareness and Competency

PC is frequently the first point of contact for patients in a health care system. As a result, PC teams work with diverse populations in terms of age, race, ethnicity, gender, sexual orientation, nationality, immigration status, and religion. These factors, which fall under the umbrella of *cultural diversity*, have been increasingly recognized as critical to the treatment of patients, due to their impact on health behaviors that confer risk for the development of health problems.

Some providers seek to incorporate issues of cultural diversity, with the goal of becoming *culturally competent* in their treatment of patients. A culturally competent approach emphasizes acquisition of knowledge and skills to treat individuals from a particular cultural background or identity, such as patients who associate with a specific religion or ethnicity. Some have questioned whether becoming a "culturally competent" provider is feasible, given the high number of cultural factors that can apply to patients. Further, there is concern that the application of information and skills that are acquired through a cultural competency approach may not apply to every individual who identifies with any given cultural factor, which may lead to stereotyping patients.

The "cultural humility" approach involves providers inviting patients to help them understand their cultural factors

In response to these concerns, health care providers are increasingly promoting the implementation of *cultural humility* when treating patients. Humility, curiosity, and sensitivity are highly emphasized in this approach. Patients are viewed as the experts in themselves and their life experiences, and providers aim to empathize, when possible, with their patient's descriptions of how elements of cultural diversity are impacting their lives. In general, a cultural humility approach can be used with every patient. Approaching patients with a collaborative energy and curiosity to understand how their unique blend of identities impact their life and health behaviors enables providers to avoid the pitfalls of assumptions that may occur when using the culturally competent approach.

Although the cultural competent approach has received extensive criticism, it is important to note that it can be used in conjunction with the cultural humility approach. The cultural competent approach may be especially helpful to providers who routinely provide services to patients who have specific cultural factors, such as patients from a certain national origin, religion, or ethnicity. Experiential learning such as attending community events that are held by members of an ethnic group that one frequently works with can be especially helpful. This information can subsequently be incorporated with the cultural humility approach, which promotes understanding of the patient's own perspectives about how any given cultural factor influences their lives.

4.6.2 Diversity, Equity, and Inclusion (DEI)

Diversity, equity, and inclusion (DEI) promote fair treatment, especially for historically underserved groups

Diversity, equity, and inclusion (DEI) refers to a conceptual framework that promotes the fair treatment of all individuals, in particular those who have been historically underserved and discriminated against. The *diversity* component of the framework emphasizes the acceptance of individuals from all backgrounds including ethnicity, gender, race, age, disability, sexual orientation, etc. *Equity* involves ensuring that everyone receives equal access to care and resources to promote their well-being. *Inclusion* refers to embracing the differences of all individuals including their perspectives and experiences. As previously described, individuals from all backgrounds receive care in PC clinics. Accordingly, adherence to the spirit and principles of DEI is critical to best serve the individuals who seek help in a PC setting.

BHPs receive training in DEI in their training programs and are often required to receive continued training in DEI by their state licensure boards. This enhances their ability to play a central role in promoting DEI in primary care clinics. Conference presentations and workshops that include elements of DEI can be especially helpful for BHPs seeking to stay up-to-date with the latest research on DEI and guidance on how to best support DEI in their PC clinic. In addition, seeking mentorship from more experienced colleagues across the country who work in PC and play a role in the implementation of DEI in their clinics can provide BHPs with invaluable information and tips.

Discussing and promoting DEI can be rewarding for BHPs who operate in PC settings, but these efforts can also be very draining. A BHP can provide their clinic staff with a lecture or workshop on DEI and have a mostly captive and participating audience, yet what they may remember the most on their commute to their home is the one colleague who clearly did not want to participate. Discussing DEI with members of a PC team can bring up divisive comments and hateful responses; undoubtedly this will impact the BHP. Attempting to maintain composure and openness to explore the thoughts of colleagues can be instrumental in managing the difficult conversations that come up when discussing DEI.

Some BHPs may have identities or be part of communities that have experienced underservice and discrimination. For these BHPs, discussing DEI factors with PC team members can potentially trigger distressing emotions, at times related to past traumas. In such cases, it is important that BHPs take some time to process whether they can lead DEI initiatives in their department and what elements of their identities and background they feel they can disclose and discuss with colleagues. Importantly, promoting DEI should be an effort that *all* members of a PC clinic champion, and the weight of promoting DEI should not fall only on the shoulders of BHPs. Moreover, leadership in the PC clinic must demonstrate a strong commitment to DEI and be mindful of not placing the responsibility on only the BHPs or other staff who are not part of the majority population.

4.6.3 Lack of Fluency With English and Use of Translators

Accurate and precise communication is critical in health care settings. As time progresses, patients who are not fluent in English are becoming increasingly likely to seek medical care in PC settings. In such situations, it is critical that they are provided with appropriate translation services that can support their ability to communicate with their providers to ensure health equity. Each PC clinic is going to have different access to translation services, and it is important to recognize that many languages have several dialects; therefore, even with translation services, the potential for miscommunications remains high. Most common translation resources involve the use of a "cart" that has a monitor in which a person will appear who can provide the translation services. Other times, there may be a telephone service that is used, or an actual person who is translating will be present in the patient room. If possible, coordination before working with a translator can ensure that encounters with patients who are not fluent in English can run smoothly. For example, identification of non-fluent-English speakers in one's schedule can prompt the acquisition of a translation cart, notification to the translator of when their services will be needed, and if possible, modification of the provider schedule, given that working with translators tends to lead to longer sessions.

Extra time may be required when translators are necessary with patients who do not speak or understand English

When working with non-fluent-English-speaking patients, it is often the case that family members or friends who accompany the patient will volunteer to translate. In general, this kind of setup is not recommended. Providing translation services requires extensive training and expertise, especially as it pertains to discussion of medical issues such as organs, physical health symptoms, medications, and medical history information. Relying on a family member to provide the translation services may lead to miscommunication between the provider and patient that can have significant negative consequences for the health of the patient. Additionally, a provider can have more assurance that the channels of communication between themselves and the patient are more accurate when using the services of a translator, given the unbiased relationship that the translator will have with everyone in the encounter.

When working with translators, it is critical that providers maintain their focus on the patient

Providers can easily begin to treat the translator as if they were the patient, and this can negatively impact rapport with the patient. Despite hearing information from the translator, it is important that providers speak to the patient. Where people are present in the room is also important, and will be influenced by the space and structure of a room. The translator should be to the side of the direct path between the provider and the patient. This can ensure that the translator is not taking up the spotlight of the encounter, which should be on the patient.

5

Case Vignettes: A Day in the Life of an Integrated Primary Care Psychologist

Primary Care Behavioral Health (PCBH) Model

7:45–10:45 a.m.	Dr. Jones, as part of their role as a behavioral health provider (BHP), provides behavioral health services for the Interdisciplinary Intensive Diabetes Clinic. This treatment team treats patients referred by their primary care provider (PCP) with a hemoglobin A1c (HbA1c) above 8.5. The treatment team consists of a physician, pharmacist, dietitian, and BHP, and various trainees from these specialties. The team provides a consultation to the PCP by working with the patient to identify steps to take to manage their diabetes and then refers the patient back to their PCP after improvements are obtained. Nine patients are scheduled typically over the course of the clinic. The clinic starts with a team huddle, followed by providers seeing different patients simultaneously for improved workflow (i.e., the dietitian is seeing patient A, the pharmacist is seeing patient B, a psychologist is seeing patient C, and a physician is seeing patient D, all at the same time). Providers then rotate through this sequence with patients. The BHP spends approximately 15 minutes with each patient. After each patient encounter, the BHP reports back to the team and enters a brief note into the electronic medical record.
7:45 a.m.	Team huddle.
8 a.m.	First visit by patient: 51-year-old man newly diagnosed with diabetes is screened with the PHQ-9 and GAD-7 (both negative); Discussions of patient's response to diagnosis; Provision of psychoeducation regarding lifestyle changes that diabetes requires and offer resources for adherence to lifestyle for diabetes; Motivational interviewing to improve patient commitment; Charting.
8:15 a.m.	First visit by patient: 62-year-old woman with history of diabetes diagnosis for over a decade is screened with the

	PHQ-9 (positive, no suicidal ideation) and GAD-7 (negative); Discussion of impact of mood on diabetes management; Activities for behavioral activation identified; Offered appointment with the Behavioral Health Clinic for follow-up but patient declines at this time; Charting.
8:30 a.m.	Return visit by patient: Fourth visit for a 47-year-old man who has not had significant changes in his HbA1c since participating in the clinic; Diabetes Distress Scale administered; Discussion of areas that are creating the greatest challenges regarding diabetes management and problem-solve about paths for improvement; Charting.
8:45 a.m.	Last visit by patient: 55-year-old woman comes for her fourth visit after notable improvements in her HbA1c: Changes made are reinforced and relapse prevention is the focus; Charting.
9:00 a.m.	Patient no show; Catch up on charting that is incomplete.
9:15 a.m.	Return visit by patient: 73-year-old woman with longstanding history of diabetes comes for her second session; Discussion of the impact of grief on her diabetes management given that her spouse died 6 months earlier; Offer grief counseling and schedule the patient for a follow-up outpatient appointment in the Behavioral Health Clinic; Charting.
9:45 a.m.	First visit by patient: 32-year-old woman who struggles with both morbid obesity and diabetes; Screen with PHQ-9 (negative) and GAD-7 (positive); Paced breathing and progressive muscle relaxation is taught; Discussion of patient's goals regarding weight and diabetes management; Charting.
10 a.m.	Patient no show: Catch up on charting that is incomplete.
10:15 a.m.	Return visit by patient: 68-year-old man comes for third visit; Alcohol use disorder is comorbid with diabetes; Motivational interviewing for reducing alcohol use to improve diabetes; Charting.
10:30 a.m.	Team wrap-up.
10:30–11:30 a.m.	Supervision with psychology graduate students and interns who are training at the Interdisciplinary Intensive Diabetes Clinic.
11:30–12:15 p.m.	Lunch.
12:15–1 p.m.	Quality improvement team meeting.

1–1:50 p.m.	Diagnostic evaluation of a 33-year-old man who has been previously diagnosed with bipolar I disorder and borderline personality disorder. The patient was seen 3 weeks ago by their PCP for a new patient visit. The patient has been referred to the psychiatry department, which has a waitlist. Therefore, the PCP has requested that the behavioral health provider follow up with the patient until a transfer of care can be made.
1:50–2:20 p.m.	Return in-person patient visit with a 37-year-old woman with ADHD. Patient's PC has prescribed the patient's medication for ADHD, and therapy focuses on teaching the patient strategies for managing her ADHD more effectively.
2:20–2:50 p.m.	Return patient video visit with a 54-year-old man who is struggling with anxiety and family stressors.
2:50–3:10 p.m.	Warm handoff with a 21-year-old woman who presents to her PCP in distress after an ER visit following panic attacks secondary to a recent choking incident. The patient is calmed by the BHP through a paced breathing exercise and then provided education about anxiety and panic attacks. CBT is introduced and a follow-up appointment with the behavioral health division is scheduled. PCP provides a prescription for a 1-week supply of medication to reduce anxiety.
3:10–3:30 p.m.	(Appointment starts 10 minutes late due to warm handoff): Return telephone visit with a 72-year-old woman whose spouse recently died.
3:30–4 p.m.	Didactic for the family medicine residents on motivational interviewing.
4–4:30 p.m.	Meeting with a first-year family medicine resident who has been placed on a performance improvement plan secondary to concerns about his medical knowledge base and professionalism.
4:30–5 p.m.	Charting.

Collaborative Care Model (CoCM): Case Manager

7:30–8 a.m.	Review the clinic's registry.
8–8:30 a.m.	Attend primary care provider (PCP) meeting and highlight patients who have previously been identified from the registry who would benefit from being referred for CoCM.

8:30–9 a.m.	Meet with Dr. Smith, a new PCP to the clinic, to discuss CoCM and how the model works, including the most efficient way for Dr. Smith to make referrals.
9 a.m.–12 p.m.	Engage in case management by reaching out by telephone and video to CoCM patients.
9–10 a.m.	Contact patients who have been identified as good candidates for CoCM and explain the CoCM model and how it would benefit them; enroll those who express an interest in participating.
10–11 a.m.	Contact a new patient, a 46-year-old woman who enrolled in CoCM to treat persistent depressive disorder, and complete an assessment (including administering the PHQ-9 and GAD-7); Assessment includes primary symptoms; stressors; current and past psychiatric pharmacological and nonpharmacological interventions; substance use assessment; risk assessment; sleep and pain assessment; medical history; family history, social history; assessment; and plan.
11 a.m.–12 p.m.	Contact a 33-year-old man who enrolled in CoCM for management of his schizoaffective disorder because he refuses to be seen in psychiatry, and complete an assessment. (The assessment includes the same items as above)
12–12:30 p.m.	Documentation of case management time and progress notes for clinical activities.
12:30–1 p.m.	Lunch.
1–2 p.m.	Meet with the CoCM team, consisting of three CoCM case managers and Dr. Smith, a psychiatrist, to discuss CoCM clinical cases.
2–4 p.m.	Engage in case management by reaching out by telephone and video to CoCM patients.
2–2:20 p.m.	Follow-up appointment with a 44-year-old woman with generalized anxiety disorder; Monitored status and provides resources.
2:20–2:35 p.m.	Follow-up appointment with a 52-year-old man with PTSD; Monitored status and provides resources.
2:35–3 p.m.	Follow-up appointment with a 66-year-old man with chronic pain and recurrent major depressive; Monitored status and provides resources.
3–3:15 p.m.	Follow-up appointment with a 33-year-old woman with panic disorder with agoraphobia; Monitored status and provides resources.
3:15–3:30 p.m.	Coordinate care with above patient's therapist.
3:30–3:40 p.m.	Follow-up appointment with a 48-year-old woman with recurrent major depressive disorder who has responded well to CoCM; End CoCM.

3:40–4 p.m.	Follow-up appointment with a 26-year-old woman with recurrent major depressive disorder; Monitored status and provides resources.
4–4:30 p.m.	Documentation of case management time and activities.

Primary Care-Mental Health Integration (PC-MHI) Model

The schedule for the day for the primary care psychologist will look like a hybrid of those for the primary care behavioral health (PCBH) model and collaborative care model (CoCM).

8–10 a.m.	The behavioral health provider (BHP) is in the PC clinic as part of the patient aligned care team (PACT) and completes five warm handoffs for veterans who need to be screened for depression and anxiety.
10–11 a.m.	Group therapy for eight veterans dealing with PTSD.
11–12 p.m.	Engage in case management by reaching out by telephone and video to CoCM patients.
11–11:30 a.m.	Contact a new patient: a 26-year-old woman who enrolled in CoCM to treat social anxiety disorder, and complete an assessment for her (including administering the PHQ-9 and GAD-7); Assessment includes primary symptoms; stressors; current and past psychiatric pharmacological and nonpharmacological interventions; substance use assessment; risk assessment; sleep and pain assessment; medical history; family history, social history; assessment; and plan.
11:30 a.m.–12 p.m.	Contact a 42-year-old man who enrolled in CoCM for management of his alcohol use disorder because he refuses to be seen in the substance abuse clinic. and complete an assessment; Engage in motivational interviewing. (The assessment includes the same items as above)
12–12:30 p.m.	Lunch.
12:30–1 p.m.	Documentation of morning's activities.
1–2 p.m.	Meet with the CoCM team, consisting of three CoCM case managers and Dr. Jones, a psychiatrist, to discuss CoCM clinical cases.
2–4 p.m.	Individual therapy appointments for 3 patients.
4–4:30 p.m.	Documentation of the afternoon's activities.

6

Further Reading

Hunter, C. L., Goodie, J. L., Oordt, M. S., & Dobmeyer, A. C. (2024). *Integrated behavioral health in primary care: Step-by-step guidance for assessment and intervention.* American Psychological Association. https://doi.org/10.1037/0000380-000
This book provides a comprehensive overview of integrated primary care. Readers are introduced to practical tools and scripts that can enhance their effectiveness in primary care settings.

McDaniel, S. H., & Ruddy, N. B. (2024). *A systematic approach to behavioral healthcare integration: Context matters.* American Psychological Association.
This book provides insights about the many challenges regarding integrating behavioral health services into medical settings and outlines various strategies for doing so successfully across multiple types of settings.

Robinson, P. J., Gould, D. A., & Strosahl, K. D. (2015). *Real behavior change in primary care: Improving patient outcomes and increasing job satisfaction.* New Harbinger.
This book introduces readers to health behavior change interventions that can be implemented in 10 minutes. The interventions are based on principles of acceptance and commitment therapy (ACT), and thus this book will be especially appealing for readers who work in integrated primary care settings and use ACT in their practices.

Robinson, P., & Reiter, J. T. (2025). *Behavioral consultation and primary care: A guide to integrating services* (3rd ed.). Springer. https://doi.org/10.1007/978-3-031-72150-2
The third edition of this book provides an updated overview of integrated care including recent developments that are impacting integration in healthcare. It provides guidance on how to promote integration across a variety of settings and thus is a helpful resource for those looking to promote integration in their facility.

Ward-Zimmerman, B., Gunn, W. B., Ruddy, N., Vogel, M. E., Cubic, B. A., Kearney, L. A., Neumann, C., Stillman, M. A., & Wells, S. (2017). *Integrated primary care psychology: An introductory curriculum.* Society for Health Psychology. https://societyforhealthpsychology.org/articles-resources/education-training/integrated-primary-care-an-introductory-curriculum/
This resource is a training curriculum based on the most up to date research related to IPC that provides foundational and topic modules related to IPC with multiple illustration, videos, interactive exercises (for more details see section on Didactic Resources in Section 4.2.4 and Tables 1 and 2).

7

References

Accreditation Council for Graduate Medical Education. (2023). *ACGME program requirements for graduate medical education.* https://www.acgme.org/specialties/family-medicine/program-requirements-and-faqs-and-applications/

Agency for Healthcare Research and Quality. (2013). *Atlas of integrated behavioral health care quality measures.* https://integrationacademy.ahrq.gov/sites/default/files/2021-09/ibhc_atlas_framework_and_measures.pdf?_gl=1*1lytqkh*_ga*NzclNzMwOTY1LjE3MzY2MzgzMDc.*_ga_45NDTD15CJ*MTczODM0Mzk5OS4xLjAuMTczODM0Mzk5OS42MC4wLjA

Ahad, A. A., Sanchez-Gonzales, M., & Junquera, P. (2023). Understanding and addressing mental health stigma across cultures for improving psychiatric care: A narrative review. *Cureus, 15*(5), Article e39549. https://doi.org/10.7759/cureus.39549

AIMS Center. (2024). *Improving population health by advancing effective integrated care.* https://aims.uw.edu/

American Medical Association. (2017). *Code of medical ethics.* https://code-medical-ethics.ama-assn.org/

American Psychiatric Association & Academy of Psychosomatic Medicine. (2016). *Dissemination of integrated care within adult primary care settings: Collaborative Care Model.*

American Psychiatric Association. (2022). *Diagnostic and statistical manual of mental disorders* (5th ed., text rev.). https://doi.org/10.1176/appi.books.9780890425787

American Psychological Association. (2017). *Ethical principles of psychologists and code of conduct: Including 2010 amendments.* http://www.apa.org/ethics/code/

American Psychological Association. (2012). Guidelines for the evaluation of dementia and age-related cognitive changes. *American Psychologist, 67*(1), 1–9. https://doi.org/10.1037/a0024643

Archer, J., Bower, P., Gilbody, S., Lovell, K., Richards, D., Gask, L., Dickens, C., & Coventry, P. (2012). Collaborative care for depression and anxiety problems. *Cochrane Database of Systematic Reviews, 10*(10), CD006525. https://doi.org/10.1002/14651858.CD006525.pub2

Beck, A. T., Rush, A. J., Shaw, B. F., Emery, G., DeRubeis, R. J., & Hollon, S. D. (2024). *Cognitive therapy of depression* (2nd ed.). Guilford.

Beehler, G. P., Verile, M., Conrad, M., & Moskal, D. (2024). Brief behavioral intervention for chronic pain in integrated primary care: What are we waiting for? [Editorial]. *Families, Systems, & Health, 42*(2), 151–156. https://doi.org/10.1037/fsh0000899

Berwick, D. M., Nolan, T. W., & Whittington, J. (2008). The triple aim: Care, health, and cost. *Health Affairs, 27*(3), 759–769. https://doi.org/10.1377/hlthaff.27.3.759

Bluestein, D., & Cubic, B. A. (2009). Psychologists and primary care physicians: A training model for creating collaborative relationships. *Journal of Clinical Psychology in Medical Settings, 16*(1), 101–112. https://doi.org/10.1007/s10880-009-9156-9

Bodenheimer, T., & Sinsky, C. (2014). From the triple to the quadruple aim: Care of the patient requires care of the provider. *Annals of Family Medicine, 12*(6), 573-576. https://doi.org/10.1370/afm.1713

Bryant, C., Bei, B., Gilson, K., Komiti, A., Jackson, H., & Judd, F. (2012). The relationship between attitudes to aging and physical and mental health in older adults.

International Psychogeriatrics, 24, 1674–1683. https://doi.org/10.1017/S1041610212000774

Burns, D. D. (1999). *Feeling good: The new mood therapy* (rev. and updated). Avon Books.

Centers for Disease Control and Prevention. (2024). *YRBS data summary & trends report*. https://www.cdc.gov/yrbs/dstr/

Chien, A. T., Leyenaar, J., Tomaino, M., Woloshin, S., Leininger, L., Barnett, E. R., McLaren, J. L., & Meara, E. (2022). Difficulty obtaining behavioral health services for children: A national survey of multiphysician practices. *Annals of Family Medicine, 20*(1), 42–50. https://doi.org/10.1370/afm.2759

Cheung, J. M. Y., Jarrin, D. C., Ballot, O., Bharwani, A. A., & Morin, C. M. (2019). A systematic review of cognitive behavioral therapy for insomnia implemented in primary care and community settings. *Sleep Medicine Reviews, 44*, 23–36. https://doi.org/10.1016/j.smrv.2018.11.001

Cubic, B. A. (2019). Consultations in medical settings. In C. Falender & E. Shafranske (Eds.), *Consultation in health service psychology: A competency-based approach* (pp. 151–168). American Psychological Association.

Cubic, B. A., & Beacham, A. O. (2014). Creating educational and training opportunities for psychology trainees in integrated care. In C. M. Hunter, C. L. Hunter, & R. S. Kessler, (Eds.), *Handbook of clinical psychology in medical settings: Evidence based assessment and intervention* (pp. 41–76). Springer.

Cubic, B. A., Neumann, C., Kearney, L., McGrath, R., Ruddy, N., Rybarczyk, B., & Zamudio, A. (2011). *Report of the Primary Care Training Taskforce to the APA Board of Educational Affairs*. American Psychological Association.

Cubic, B. A., Mance, J., Turgesen, J. N., & Lamanna, J. D. (2012). Interprofessional education: Preparing psychologists for success in integrated care. *Journal of Clinical Psychology in Medical Settings, 19*, 84–92. https://doi.org/10.1007/s10880-011-9291-y

Cummings, N. A., O'Donohue, W., Hays, S. C., & Follette, V. (2001). *Integrated behavioral healthcare: Positioning mental health practice with medical/surgical practice*. Academic Press.

Davidson, J. R., Dickson, C., & Han, H. (2019). Cognitive behavioural treatment for insomnia in primary care: A systematic review of sleep outcomes. *British Journal of General Practice: Journal of the Royal College of General Practitioners, 69*(686), e657–e664. https://doi.org/10.3399/bjgp19X705065

Elshaikh, U., Sheik, R., Saeed, R. K. M., Chivese, T., & Alsayed Hassan, D. (2023). Barriers and facilitators of older adults for professional mental health help-seeking: A systematic review. *BMC Geriatrics, 23*(1), Article 516. https://doi.org/10.1186/s12877-023-04229-x

English, I., Cameron, J. J., & Campbell, D. G. (2024). Degree of primary care integration predicts job satisfaction and emotional exhaustion among rural medical and behavioral healthcare providers. *Families, Systems, & Health, 42*(3), 375–379. https://doi.org/10.1037/fsh0000905

Espie, C. A. (2002). Insomnia: Conceptual issues in the development, persistence, and treatment of sleep disorder in adults. *Annual Review of Psychology, 53*, 215–243. https://doi.org/10.1146/annurev.psych.53.100901.135243

Foa, E. B., Hembree, E. A., & Rothbaum, B. O. (2007). *Prolonged exposure therapy for PTSD: Emotional processing of traumatic experiences: Therapist guide*. Oxford University Press. https://doi.org/10.1093/med:psych/9780195308501.001.0001

Francesco, P., Mauro, M. G., Gianluca, C., & Enrico, M. (2010). The efficacy of relaxation training in treating anxiety. *International Journal of Behavioral Consultation and Therapy, 5*(3-4), 264–269. https://doi.org/10.1037/h0100887

Fraser, M. W., Lombardi, B. M., Wu, S., Zerden, L. S. Richman, E. L., & Fraher, E. P. (2018). Integrated primary care and social work: A systematic review. *Journal of the Society for Social Work and Research, 9*, 175–215. https://doi.org/10.1086/697567

Friedman, D. (1978). Academic family medicine. *JAMA, 240*(23), 2539–2540. https://doi.org/10.1001/jama.1978.03290230031011

Funderburk, J. S., Wray, L. O., Martin, J., & Maisto, S. A. (2024). How do models of integrated primary care work? A proposed model for mechanisms of change using primary care behavioral health. *Psychological Services, 21*(3), 569–580. https://doi.org/10.1037/ser0000871

Gass, J. C., Maisto, S. A., Edelman, D., & Funderburk, J. S. (2023). Brief conjoint visits between an embedded behavioral health provider and primary care team member: When are they used and what are the barriers and facilitators? *Families, Systems, & Health, 41*(4), 488–501. https://doi.org/10.1037/fsh0000817

Gotlieb, E. M., Cotsonis, G. A., Magill, M., Gotlieb, J., Marcus, S., Patterson, K., Spandorfer, P., Tim, M., Yedvobnick, L., & Douglas, B. (2014). The time burden for pediatricians caring for adolescents with behavioral issues. *Journal of Adolescent Health, 54*(Suppl), S70. https://doi.org/10.1016/j.jadohealth.2013.10.153

Graziano, P. A., Ros-Demarize, R., & Hare, M. M. (2020). Condensing parent training: A randomized trial comparing the efficacy of a briefer, more intensive version of Parent-Child Interaction Therapy (I-PCIT). *Journal of Consulting and Clinical Psychology, 88*(7), 669–679. https://doi.org/10.1037/ccp0000504

Green, L. A., Miller, W. L., Frey, J. J., Jason, H., Westberg, J., Cohen, D. J., Gotler, R. S., & DeGry, F. V. (2022). The time is now: A plan to redesign family medicine residency education. *Family Medicine, 54* (1), 7–15. https://doi.org/10.22454/FamMed.2022.197486

Gual-Montolio, P., Jaén, I., Martínez-Borba, V., Castilla, D., & Suso-Ribera, C. (2022). Using artificial intelligence to enhance ongoing psychological interventions for emotional problems in real- or close to real-time: A systematic review. *International Journal of Environmental Research and Public Health, 19*(13), Article 7737. https://doi.org/10.3390/ijerph19137737

Gunn, W. B., Jr. (2024). Review of Connections in the Clinic: Relational Narratives From Team-Based Primary Care. *Families, Systems, & Health, 42*(2), 278–279. https://doi.org/10.1037/fsh0000866

Hargraves, D., White, C., Frederick, R., Cinibulk, M., Peters, M., Young, A., & Elder, N. (2017). Implementing SBIRT (Screening, Brief Intervention and Referral to Treatment) in primary care: Lessons learned from a multi-practice evaluation portfolio. *Public Health Reviews, 38*, Article 31. https://doi.org/10.1186/s40985-017-0077-0

Hayes, S. C., Strosahl, K. D., & Wilson, K. G. (1999). *Acceptance and commitment therapy: An experiential approach to behavior change.* Guilford Press.

Health Resources and Services Administration. (2024). *State of the U.S. health care workforce.* https://bhw.hrsa.gov/sites/default/files/bureau-health-workforce/state-of-the-health-workforce-report-2024.pdf

Hoge, M. A., Morris, J. A., Laraia, M., Pomerantz, A., & Farley, T. (2014). *Core competencies for integrated behavioral health and primary care.* SAMSHA-HRSA Center for Integrated Health Solutions.

Hopper, S. I., Murray, S. L., Ferrara, L. R., & Singleton, J. K. (2019). Effectiveness of diaphragmatic breathing for reducing physiological and psychological stress in adults: A quantitative systematic review. *JBI Database of Systematic Reviews and Implementation Reports, 17*(9), 1855–1876. https://doi.org/10.11124/JBISRIR-2017-003848

Huffstetler, A., & Topmiller, M. (2024). Primary care access in areas of the United States with aging populations. *American Family Physician, 109*(4), 308–309.

Hughes, P. M., Annis, I. E., McGrath, R. E., & Thomas, K. C. (2024). *Psychotropic medication prescribing across medical providers*, 2016–2019. *Psychiatric Services, 75*(5), 477–480. https://doi.org/10.1176/appi.ps.20230156

Hunter, C. L, Funderburk, J. S., Polaha, J., Bauman, D., Goodie, J. L., & Hunter, C. M. (2018). Primary Care Behavioral Health (PCBH) model research: Current state of the science and a call to action. *Journal of Clinical Psychology in Medical Settings, 25*, 127–156. https://doi.org/10.1007/s10880-017-9512-0

Hunter, C. L., Goodie, J. L., Oordt, M. S., & Dobmeyer, A. C. (2024). *Integrated behavioral health in primary care: Step-by-step guidance for assessment and intervention.* American Psychological Association. https://doi.org/10.1037/0000380-000

Institute of Medicine, Committee on the Future of Primary Care. (1994). *Defining primary care: An interim report.* National Academy Press.

Interprofessional Education Collaborative. (2023). *IPEC core competencies for interprofessional collaborative practice: Version 3.* https://www.ipecollaborative.org/assets/core-competencies/IPEC_Core_Competencies_Version_3_2023.pdf

Jerath, R., Crawford, M. W., Barnes, V. A., & Harden, K. (2015). Self-regulation of breathing as a primary treatment for anxiety. *Applied Psychophysiology and Biofeedback, 40*(2), 107–115. https://doi.org/10.1007/s10484-015-9279-8

Johnson, J. G., Harris, E. S., Spitzer, R. L., & Williams, J. B. W. (2002). The Patient Health Questionnaire for Adolescents: Validation of an instrument for the assessment of mental disorders among adolescent primary care patients. *Journal of Adolescent Health, 30*, 196–204. https://doi.org/10.1016/s1054-139x(01)00333-0

Kiernan, R. J., Mueller, J., & Langston, J. W. (1995). *Cognistat (Neurobehavioral Cognitive Status Examination)*. Psychological Assessment Resources.

Koehler, A. N., Trejo, G., Sandberg, J. C., Swain, B. H., Marion, G. S., & Kirk, J. K. (2020). Patient views of behavioral health providers in primary care: A qualitative study of 2 southeastern clinics. *Journal of Patient Experience, 7*(4), 527–533. https://doi.org/10.1177/2374373519860357

Kovacs, M., (1985). The Children's Depression Inventory (CDI). *Psychopharmacology Bulletin, 21*, 995–998.

Kroenke, K., Spitzer, R. L., & Williams, J. B. W. (2001). The PHQ-9: Validity of a brief depression severity measure. *Journal of General Internal Medicine, 16*, 606–613. https://doi.org/10.1046/j.1525-1497.2001.016009606.x

Laborde, S., Allen, M. S., Borges, U., Dosseville, F., Hosang, T. J., Iskra, M., Mosley, E., Salvotti, C., Spolverato, L., Zammit, N., & Javelle, F. (2022). Effects of voluntary slow breathing on heart rate and heart rate variability: A systematic review and a meta-analysis. *Neuroscience and Biobehavioral Reviews, 138*, Article 104711. https://doi.org/10.1016/j.neubiorev.2022.104711

Lang, A. J. (2005). Mental health treatment preferences of primary care patients. *Journal of Behavioral Medicine, 28*, 581–586. https://doi.org/10.1007/s10865-005-9019-2

Lehrer, P. M., Woolfolk, R. L., & Sime, W. E. (Eds.). (2007). *Principles and practice of stress management* (3rd ed.). Guilford Press.

Lester, T. R., Herrmann, J. E., Bannett, Y., Gardner, R. M., Feldman, H. M., & Huffman, L. C. (2023). Anxiety and depression treatment in primary care pediatrics. *Pediatrics, 151*(5), Article e2022058846. https://doi.org/10.1542/peds.2022-058846

Levy, S. R., Slade, M. D., Murphy, T. E., & Gill, T. M. (2012). Association between positive age stereotypes and recovery from disability in older persons. *JAMA, 308*, 1972–1973. https://doi.org/10.1001/jama.2012.14541

Lieneman, C. C., Brabson, L. A., Highlander, A., Wallace, N. M., & McNeil, C. B. (2017). Parent-child interaction therapy: Current perspectives. *Psychology Research and Behavior Management, 10*, 239–256. https://doi.org/10.2147/PRBM.S91200

Ma, K. P. K., Mollis, B. L., Rolfes, J., Au, M., Crocker, A., Scholle, S. H., Kessler, R., Baldwin, L. M., & Stephens, K. A. (2022). Payment strategies for behavioral health integration in hospital-affiliated and non-hospital-affiliated primary care practices. *Translational Behavioral Medicine, 12*(8), 878–883. https://doi.org/10.1093/tbm/ibac053

Mauer, B. (2006). *Behavioral health/primary care integration: The Four Quadrant Model and evidence-based practices.* National Council for Community Behavioral Healthcare. http://www.thenationalcouncil.org/galleries/business-practice%20files/4%20Quadrant.pdf/

Mauer, B. J., & Jarvis, D. (2010). *The business case for bidirectional integrated care: Mental health and substance use services in primary care settings and primary care services in specialty mental health and substance use settings.* https://archive.thepcc.org/sites/default/files/resources/CiMH%20Business%20Case%20for%20Integration%206-30-2010%20Final.pdf

McDaniel, S. H., Grus, C. L., Cubic, B. A., Hunter, C., Kearney, L., Schumann, C., Sturm, L. & the Interorganizational. Workgroup on Competencies for Primary Care Psychology. (2014). Competencies for psychology practice in primary care. *American Psychologist, 69,* 409–429. https://doi.org/10.1037/a0036072

Miller, W. R., & Rollnick, S. (2013). *Motivational interviewing: Helping people change* (3rd ed.). Guilford Press.

Mitchell, D., Olson, A., & Randolph, N. (2022). The impact of warm handoffs on patient engagement with behavioral health services in primary care. *Journal of Rural Mental Health, 46*(2), 82–87. https://doi.org/10.1037/rmh0000199

Molinari, V. (Ed.). (2011). *Specialty competencies in geropsychology.* Oxford University Press.

Moon, D. J., Damman, J. L., & Romero, A. (2020). The effects of primary care-based parenting interventions on parenting and child behavioral outcomes: A systematic review. *Trauma, Violence & Abuse, 21*(4), 706–724. https://doi.org/10.1177/1524838018774424

Muhammad Khir, S., Wan Mohd Yunus, W. M. A., Mahmud, N., Wang, R., Panatik, S. A., Mohd Sukor, M. S., & Nordin, N. A. (2024). Efficacy of progressive muscle relaxation in adults for stress, anxiety, and depression: A systematic review. *Psychology Research and Behavior Management, 17,* 345–365. https://doi.org/10.2147/PRBM.S437277

Murray, M., & Tantau, C. (2000). Same-day appointments: Exploding the access paradigm. *Family Practice Management, 7*(8), 45–50.

Nash, J. M., Khatri, P., Cubic, B. A., & Baird, M. A. (2013). Essential competencies for psychologists in patient centered medical homes. *Professional Psychology: Research and Practice, 44,* 331–342. https://doi.org/10.1037/a0033106

Nasreddine, Z. S., Phillips, N. A., Bedirian, V., Charbonneau, S., Whitehead, V., Collin, I., Cummings, J. L., & Chertkow, H. (2005). The Montreal Cognitive Assessment, MoCA: A brief screening tool for mild cognitive impairment. *Journal of American Geriatric Society, 53,* 695–699. https://doi.org/10.1111/j.1532-5415.2005.53221x

National Association of Social Workers. (2021). *Code of ethics.* https://www.socialworkers.org/About/Ethics/Code-of-Ethics/Code-of-Ethics-English

Nederveld, A., Wiggins, K., Dickinson, L. M., Dickinson, P. W., Tolle, L. W., & Holtrop, J. S. (2023). Integrated primary care and health behavior support: A survey of behavioral health providers. *Journal of Primary Care & Community Health, 14,* 21501319231172039. https://doi.org/10.1177/21501319231172039

Nezu, A. M., Maguth Nezu, C., & D'Zurilla, T. J. (2013). *Problem-solving therapy: A treatment manual.* Springer.

Peek, C. J., & National Integration Academy Council. (2013). *Lexicon for behavioral health and primary care integration: Concepts and definitions by expert consensus* (AHRQ Publication No. 13-IP001-EF). Agency for Healthcare Research and Quality https://integrationacademy.ahrq.gov/sites/default/files/2020-06/Lexicon.pdf

Possemato, K., Johnson, E. M., Beehler, G. P., Shepardson, R. L., King, P., Vair, C. L., Funderburk, J. S., Maisto, S. A., & Wray, L. O. (2018). Patient outcomes associated with primary care behavioral health services: A systematic review. *General Hospital Psychiatry, 53,* 1–11. https://doi.org/10.1016/j.genhosppsych.2018.04.002

Raffoul, M., Moore, M., Kamerow, D., & Bazemore, A. (2016). A primary care panel size of 2500is neither accurate nor reasonable. (2016). *Journal of the American Board of Family Medicine, 29*(4), 496–499. https://doi.org/10.3122/jabfm.2016.04.150317

Rameez, S., & Nasir, A. (2023). Barriers to mental health treatment in primary care practice in low- and middle-income countries in a post-COVID era. A systemic review. *Journal of Family Medicine Primary Care, 12*(8), 1485–1504. https://doi.org/10.4103/jfmpc.jfmpc_391_22

Randolph, C., Tierney, M. C., Mohr, E., & Chase, T. N. (1998). The Repeatable Battery for the Assessment of Neuropsychological Status (RBANS): Preliminary clinical validity. *Journal of Clinical and Experimental Neuropsychology, 20*, 310–319. https://doi.org/10.1076/jcen.20.3.310.823

Rauch, S. A. M., Venners, M. R., Ragin, C., Ruhe, G., Lamp, K. E., Burton, M., Pomerantz, A., Bernardy, N., Schnurr, P. P., Hamblen, J. L., Possemato, K., Sripada, R., Wray, L. O., Dollar, K., Wade, M., Astin, M. C., & Cigrang, J. A. (2023). Treatment of posttraumatic stress disorder with prolonged exposure for primary care (PE-PC): Effectiveness and patient and therapist factors related to symptom change and retention. *Psychological Services, 20*(4), 745–755. https://doi.org/10.1037/ser0000783

Reiss-Brennan, B., Brunisholz, K. D., Dredge, C., Briot, P., Grazier, K., Wilcox, A., Savitz, L., & James, B. (2016). Association of integrated team-based care with health care quality, utilization, and cost. *JAMA, 316*(8), 826–834. https://doi.org/10.1001/jama.2016.11232

Reist, C., Petiwala, I., Latimer, J., Raffaelli, S.B., Chiang, M., Eisenberg, D., & Campbell, S. (2022). Collaborative mental health care: A narrative review. *Medicine, 101*(52), Article e32554. https://doi.org/10.1097/MD.0000000000032554

Reiter, J. T., Dobmeyer, A. C., & Hunter, C. L. (2018). The Primary Care Behavioral Health (PCMH) model: An overview and operational definition. *Journal of Clinical Psychology in Medical Settings, 25*, 109–126. https://doi.org/10.1007/s10880-017-9531-x

Resick, P. A., Monson, C. M., & Chard, K. M. (2024). *Cognitive processing therapy for PTSD: A comprehensive therapist manual* (2nd ed.). Guilford Press.

Rose, G. L., Weldon, T. L., McEntee, M. L., Hitt, J. R., Kessler, R., Littenberg, B., Macchi, C. R., Martin, M. P., Mullin, D. J., & van Eeghen, C. (2023). Practice integration profile revised: Improving item readability and completion. *Families, Systems & Health, 41*, 201–206. https://doi.org/10.1037/fsh0000723

Rubin, M., Arnon, H., Huppert, J. D., & Perry, A. (2024). Considering the role of human empathy in AI-driven therapy. *JMIR Mental Health, 11*, e56529. https://doi.org/10.2196/56529

Ryan, R. M., & Deci, E. L. (2000). Self-determination theory and the facilitation of intrinsic motivation, social development, and well-being. *American Psychologist, 55*(1), 68–78. https://doi.org/10.1037/0003-066X.55.1.68

Schmidt, M. K., Watson, J. C., & Fernandez, M. A. (2018). Examining the effectiveness of integrated behavioral and primary health care treatment. *Journal of Counseling Development, 96*, 3–14. https://doi.org/10.1002/jcad.12173

Scogin, F., Rohen, N., & Bailey, E. (2000). Geriatric Depression Scale. In M. E. Maruish (Ed.), *Handbook of psychological assessment in primary care settings* (pp. 491–508). Lawrence Erlbaum.

Scott, V. C., Kenworthy, T., Godly-Reynolds, E., Bastien, G., Scaccia, J., McMickens, C., Rachel, S., Cooper, S., Wrenn, G., & Wandersman, A. (2017). The Readiness for Integrated Care Questionnaire (RICQ): An instrument to assess readiness to integrate behavioral health and primary care. *American Journal of Orthopsychiatry, 87*, 520–530. https://doi.org/10.1037/ort0000270

Serrano, N. F., Cordes, C., Cubic, B. A., & Daub, S. (2017). The state and future of primary care behavioral health workforce. *Journal of Clinical Psychology in Medical Settings, 24*, 157–168. https://doi.org/10.1007/s10880-017-9491-1

Shepardson, R. L., Fletcher, T. L., Funderburk, J. S., Weisberg, R. B., Beehler, G. P., & Maisto, S. A. (2023). Barriers to and facilitators of using evidence-based, cognitive-behavioral anxiety interventions in integrated primary care practice. *Psychological Services, 20*(4), 709–722. https://doi.org/10.1037/ser0000696

Spielman, A. J., Caruso, L. S., & Glovinsky, P. B. (1987). A behavioral perspective on insomnia treatment. *Psychiatric Clinics of North America, 10*(4), 541–553. https://doi.org/10.1016/S0193-953X(18)30532-X

Spitzer, R. L., Kroenke, K., Williams, J. B. W., & Lowe, B. (2006). *Generalized Anxiety Disorder 7 (GAD-7)*. American Psychiatric Association Psychological Tests. https://doi.org/10.1037/t02591-000

Stillman, M. A., Mullen, C. M., Grosse, C. V., & Hewitt, K. C. (2018). Preliminary analysis of an innovative curriculum in integrated primary care psychology: Assessment of student interest and competency. *Journal of Psychiatry and Behavioral Sciences, 1*, 1–8. https://doi.org/10.33582/2637-8027/1001

Sturgeon J. A. (2014). Psychological therapies for the management of chronic pain. *Psychology Research and Behavior Management, 7*, 115–124. https://doi.org/10.2147/PRBM.S44762

Sultzer, D. L. (1994). Mental status examination. In C. E. Coffey, J. L. Cummings, M. R. Lovell, & G. D. Pearlson (Eds.). *The American Psychiatric Press textbook of geriatric neuropsychiatry* (pp. 111–127). American Psychiatric Association.

U.S. Centers for Medicare & Medical Services. (2024). *Resources for Integrated Care: Behavioral Health Integration Capacity Assessment*. https://www.cms.gov/files/zip/ricresource-behavioralhealthintegrationcapacityassessment.zip

Ward-Zimmerman, B., Gunn, W. B., Ruddy, N., Vogel, M. E., Cubic, B. A., Kearney, L. A., Neumann, C., Stillman, M. A., & Wells, S. (2017). *Integrated primary care psychology: An introductory curriculum*. Society for Health Psychology. https://societyforhealthpsychology.org.training/integrated-primary-care-psychology/

Weathers, F. W., Litz, B. T., Keane, T. M., Palmieri, P. A., Marx, B. P., & Schnurr, P. P. (2013). *The PTSD Checklist for DSM-5 (PCL-5) - Standard* [Measurement instrument]. https//www.ptsd.gov/professional/assessment/adult-sr/ptsd-checklist.asp

Williams, P. G., Suchy, Y., & Rau, H. K. (2009). Individual differences in executive functioning: Implications for stress regulation. *Annals of Behavioral Medicine, 37*(2), 126–140. https://doi.org/10.1007/s12160-009-9100-0

Zhang, A., Park, S., Sullivan, J. E., & Jing, S. (2018). The effectiveness of problem-solving therapy for primary care patients' depressive and/or anxiety disorders: A systematic review and meta-analysis. *Journal of the American Board of Family Medicine, 31*, 139–150. https://doi.org/10.3122/jabfm.2018.01.170270

8

Appendix: Tools and Resources

The following materials for your book can be downloaded free of charge once you register on the Hogrefe website.

Appendix 1: Safety Plan
Appendix 2: Sample of Resources With Worksheets and Handouts for Patients
Appendix 3: Sample of App Resources

How to proceed:

DOWNLOAD

1. Go to www.hgf.io/media and create a user account. If you already have one, please log in.
2. Go to **My supplementary materials** in your account dashboard and enter the code below. You will automatically be redirected to the download area, where you can access and download the supplementary materials.

   Code: B-IIPEF4

To make sure you have permanent direct access to all the materials, we recommend that you download them and save them on your computer.

Appendix 1: Safety Plan

This is a **preview** of the content that is available in the downloadable material of this book. Please see p. 78 for instructions on how to obtain the full-sized, printable PDF.

Step 1 Warning signs
(What tells you that you might be most at risk for suicidal thoughts, e.g., when you haven't had contact with others for several days, when your pain level is greater than 7, when you feel hopeless about your future)

1. ______________________________
2. ______________________________
3. ______________________________

Step 2 Internal coping strategies – things I can do to take my mind off my problems without contacting another person
(e.g., write in a journal, meditate, etc.)

1. ______________________________
2. ______________________________
3. ______________________________

Step 3 People and social settings that provide distraction
(People you enjoy spending time with or places you can go to get a break from your negative thoughts)

1. Name ____________________ Phone ____________
2. Name ____________________ Phone ____________
3. Place ____________________
4. Place ____________________

Step 4 People whom I can ask for help
(e.g., individuals I trust to be compassionate and keep my concerns private)

1. Name ____________________ Phone ____________
2. Name ____________________ Phone ____________
3. Name ____________________ Phone ____________

Step 5 Professionals or agencies I can contact during a crisis

1. Clinician name ______________________ Phone: ______________
2. Clinician name ______________________ Phone: ______________
3. Clinician emergency contact number(s) ______________________
4. Local hospital ER ______________________ Phone: ______________

   Address ______________________
5. Area crisis response line phone number ______________________
6. Suicide prevention hotline Call or Text 988
7. Apps I can use: CalmHarm, Safety Net

Step 6 Making the environment safe
(Remove all weapons from the home, ask a loved one to keep your medications for a while and give them to you as needed, etc.)

1. ______________________
2. ______________________
3. ______________________

This is a **preview** of the content that is available in the downloadable material of this book. Please see p. 78 for instructions on how to obtain the full-sized, printable PDF.

Appendix 2: Sample of Resources With Worksheets and Handouts for Patients

This is a **preview** of the content that is available in the downloadable material of this book. Please see p. 78 for instructions on how to obtain the full-sized, printable PDF.

Depression

Mind over mood: Change how you feel by changing the way you think (2nd ed.).
By Dennis Greenberger and Christine A. Padesky.

Mood Regulation

DBT skills training: Handouts and worksheets.
By Marsha M. Linehan.

Trauma

Cognitive processing therapy for PTSD: A comprehensive manual (1st ed.).
By Patricia Resick, Candice Monson, and Kathleen Chard.

Prolonged exposure therapy for PTSD: Emotional processing of traumatic experiences, therapist guide (2nd ed.).
By Edna Foa, Elizabeth A. Hembree, Barbara Olasov Rothbaum, and Sheila Rauch.

Anxiety

Mastery of your anxiety and panic: Workbook for primary care settings.
By Michelle G. Craske and David H. Barlow.

Insomnia

Cognitive behavioral treatment of insomnia: A session-by-session guide.
By Michael L. Perlis, Carla Benson-Jungquist, Michael T. Smith, and Donn A. Posner.

Sleep diary PDF: https://www.uclahealth.org/sites/default/files/documents/sleepdiary.pdf

Meditation Resources (Websites, Applications)

https://www.insighttimer.com/: This website/application offers a large collection of free guided meditations and resources including blogs and videos for common mental health problems. Users of insighttimer have access to meditations that are designed to help with several areas including sleep and stress/anxiety reduction.

YouTube: Jon Kabat-Zinn meditation recordings

Dartmouth Student Wellness Center: Recordings for deep-breathing, meditation, progressive muscle relaxation. https://students.dartmouth.edu/wellness-center/wellness-mindfulness/mindfulness-meditation/guided-recordings/mindfulness-meditation

Assertive Communication

Your perfect right: Assertiveness and equality in your life and relationships (10th ed.).
By Robert Alberti and Michael Emmons.

Websites With Resources on Determining Readiness for Integration and Other Helpful Resources for Clinicians and Patients

Integrating Behavioral Health and Primary Care Playbook:
https://integrationacademy.ahrq.gov/products/playbooks/behavioral-health-and-primary-care?c-9-NIAC

Behavioral Health Integration Fact Sheet:
https://www.apa.org/health/behavioral-integration-fact-sheet

Compendium of Resources for Integrated Primary Care Providers:
https://www.ama-assn.org/public-health/behavioral-health/compendium-behavioral-health-integration-resources-physician

This is a **preview** of the content that is available in the downloadable material of this book. Please see p. 78 for instructions on how to obtain the full-sized, printable PDF.

Appendix 3: Sample of App Resources

This is a **preview** of the content that is available in the downloadable material of this book. Please see p. 78 for instructions on how to obtain the full-sized, printable PDF.

There are several apps that can be recommended to patients being seen in IPC, and more are always under development. The possibilities regarding technology-based resources will also likely continue to expand with generative AI.

In choosing to suggest apps for IPC, the BHP should download the app onto their computer, electronic notebook, or phone to be able to demonstrate the app and how it might be useful. Apps recommended should focus on ones that are easily accessible and user-friendly. Apps that assist with coping skill development (e.g., relaxation, cognitive restructuring, behavioral activation) and symptom tracking (e.g. sleep, pain, mood) are most suitable for IPC. BHPs and PCPs should reinforce use of the apps and ensure that the patient has the health literacy to use the app appropriately.

Please note that some of these apps are free, while others have a fee or a subscription charge.

Examples of commonly used apps in PC are:

Breathe2Relax (breathing skills)

Calm (relaxation skills)

Calm Harm (skills for coping with suicidal ideation)

CPT Coach (supplement for patients participating in cognitive processing therapy)

DBT Coach (skills for emotional regulation, interpersonal effectiveness, mindfulness, and distress tolerance)

Headspace (mindfulness and meditation activities)

Mindshift (skills for management of anxiety)

Moodpath (skills for mood tracking and awareness)

Noom (skills for healthy eating and lifestyle changes to achieve weight loss)

PTSD Coach (skills for management of PTSD)

Safety Net (provides direction for safety planning)

Self Help for Anxiety Management (skills for management of anxiety)

Peer Commentaries

Cubic and Tinajero deliver a pragmatic, experience-rich, and engaging guide to thriving as a behavioral health provider in integrated primary care. With clear "how-to" strategies and compassionate, evidence-based insights, they bring to life the real-world challenges and deep rewards of collaborative healthcare. A must-read for clinicians and graduate students eager to pursue impactful and fulfilling careers in integrated care.

Barbara Ward-Zimmerman, PhD, Past President, Society for Health Psychology (American Psychological Association, Division 38)

This is a concise and articulate discussion of integrated primary care that links theory with pragmatic application. A must have for psychologists interested in implementing this approach. Also, a marvelous resource for engaging trainees and sparking interest in integrated care models. Ultimate beneficiaries of Drs. Cubic's and Tinajero's work will be the myriad of patients and caregivers whose health will be promoted as a result.

Daniel Bluestein, MD, MS, CMD-R, AGSF-R, Professor Emeritus, Department of Family & Community Medicine, Eastern Virginia Medical School, Norfolk, VA

Thank you to Cubic and Tinajero for providing us with a brief, practical, and accessible description of the richness that is integrated primary care, an approach that increases access for the many patients with biopsychosocial health issues and allows us to provide care we cannot when working in silos. The authors capture the excitement involved in bringing together primary care and behavioral health professionals to team with patients and families in providing whole person, family-oriented care that is sensitive to community and cultural values. While brief, the book is comprehensive and provides a great overview for new students to the field while summarizing it for someone who is deeply embedded in it.

Susan McDaniel, PhD, Dr. Laurie Sands Distinguished Professor of Families & Health, Departments of Psychiatry and Family Medicine, University of Rochester Medical Center, Rochester, NY

This concise book will help behavioral health professionals understand the context of primary care and develop integrated behavioral health competencies related to evidence-based clinical care, clinical consultation, and practice improvement. The book helps to fill a void in resources to prepare behavioral health professionals for evolving roles in primary care.

Nancy Ruddy, PhD, Affiliate Faculty, Department of Psychology, University of Maine, Orono, ME

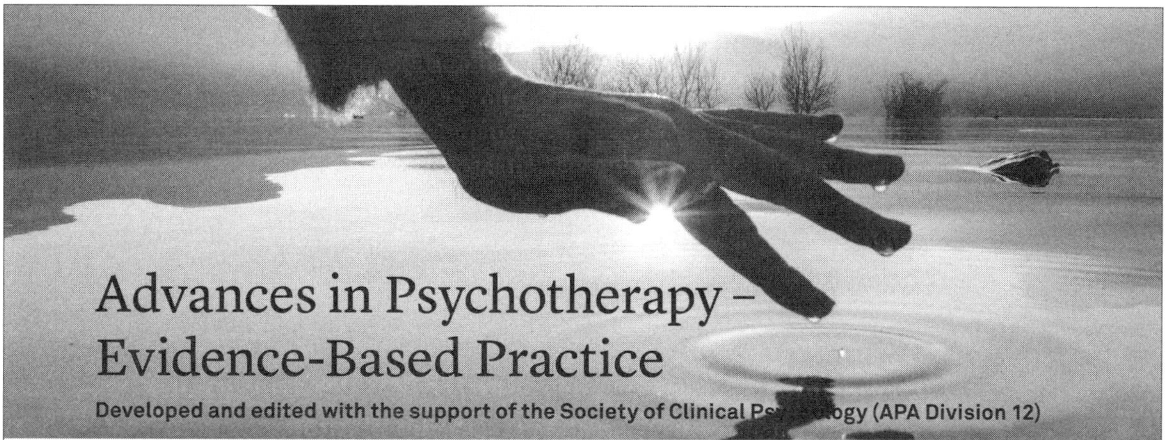

Advances in Psychotherapy – Evidence-Based Practice

Developed and edited with the support of the Society of Clinical Psychology (APA Division 12)

Series editors
J. Kim Penberthy, PhD, ABPP
Heather Bruschwein, PsyD, ABPP
Jonathan S. Comer, PhD
Damion Grasso, PhD
Sarah Meshberg-Cohen, PhD
Jonathan Weinand, PhD

- *Practice-oriented*
- *Evidence-based*
- *Expert authors*
- *Easy-to-read*
- *Compact*
- *Cost-effective*

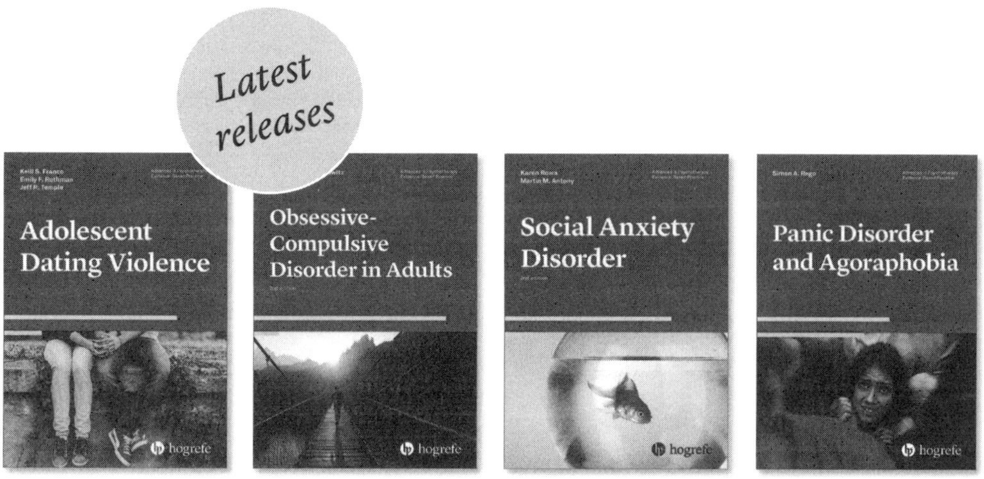

Volume 56 | Volume 31, 2nd ed. | Volume 12, 2nd ed. | Volume 55

www.hogrefe.com/apt

hogrefe

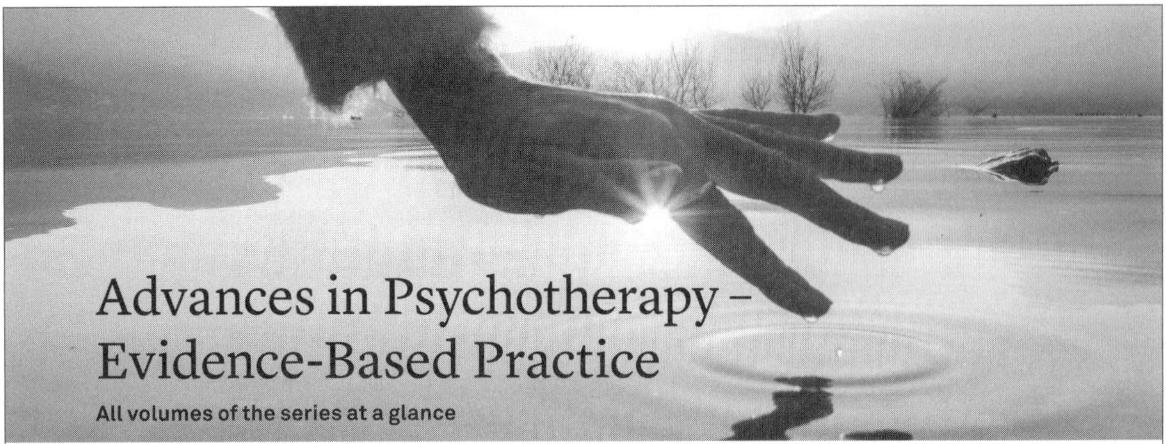

Adolescent Dating Violence (Vol. 56)
Affirmative Counseling for Transgender and Gender Diverse Clients (Vol. 45)
Alcohol Use Disorders (Vol. 10)
Alzheimer's Disease and Dementia (Vol. 38)
ADHD in Adults, 2nd ed., (Vol. 35)
ADHD in Children and Adolescents, 2nd ed. (Vol. 33)
Autism Spectrum Disorder (Vol. 29)
Binge Drinking and Alcohol Misuse Among College Students and Young Adults (Vol. 32)
Bipolar Disorder, 2nd ed. (Vol. 1)
Body Dysmorphic Disorder (Vol. 44)
Childhood Depression (Vol. 54)
Childhood Maltreatment, 2nd ed. (Vol. 4)
Childhood Obesity (Vol. 39)
Chronic Illness in Children and Adolescents (Vol. 9)
Chronic Pain (Vol. 11)
Depression (Vol. 18)
Developing Anti-Racist Cultural Competence (Vol. 53)
Eating Disorders (Vol. 13)
Elimination Disorders in Children and Adolescents (Vol. 16)
Family Caregiver Distress (Vol. 50)
Generalized Anxiety Disorder (Vol. 24)
Growing Up with Domestic Violence (Vol. 23)
Harm Reduction Treatment for Substance Use (Vol. 49)
Headache (Vol. 30)
Heart Disease (Vol. 2)
Hoarding Disorder (Vol. 40)
Hypochondriasis and Health Anxiety (Vol. 19)
Insomnia (Vol. 42)
Integrating Digital Tools into Children's Mental Health Care (Vol. 52)
Internet Addiction (Vol. 41)
Language Disorders in Children and Adolescents (Vol. 28)
Mindfulness (Vol. 37)
Multiple Sclerosis (Vol. 36)
Nicotine and Tobacco Dependence (Vol. 21)
Nonsuicidal Self-Injury (Vol. 22)
Obsessive-Compulsive Disorder in Adults, 2nd ed. (Vol. 31)
Occupational Stress (Vol. 51)
Panic Disorder and Agoraphobia (Vol. 55)
Persistent Depressive Disorders (Vol. 43)
Phobic and Anxiety Disorders in Children and Adolescents (Vol. 27)
Problem and Pathological Gambling (Vol. 8)
Psychological Approaches to Cancer Care (Vol. 46)
Public Health Tools for Practicing Psychologists (Vol. 20)
Sexual Dysfunction in Women (Vol. 25)
Sexual Dysfunction in Men (Vol. 26)
Sexual Violence (Vol. 17)
Social Anxiety Disorder, 2nd ed. (Vol. 12)
Substance Use Problems, 2nd ed. (Vol. 15)
Suicidal Behavior, 2nd ed. (Vol. 14)
The Schizophrenia Spectrum, 2nd ed. (Vol. 5)
Time-Out in Child Behavior Management (Vol. 48)
Treating Victims of Mass Disaster and Terrorism (Vol. 6)
Women and Drinking: Preventing Alcohol-Exposed Pregnancies (Vol. 34)

www.hogrefe.com/apt

hogrefe